Special Education in Context

Special Education in Context

An ethnographic study of persons
with developmental disabilities

John Joseph Gleason
Department of Special Education, Rhode Island College

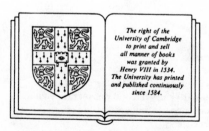

The right of the
University of Cambridge
to print and sell
all manner of books
was granted by
Henry VIII in 1534.
The University has printed
and published continuously
since 1584.

Cambridge University Press
Cambridge
New York   New Rochelle   Melbourne   Sydney

CAMBRIDGE UNIVERSITY PRESS
Cambridge, New York, Melbourne, Madrid, Cape Town, Singapore,
São Paulo, Delhi, Dubai, Tokyo

Cambridge University Press
The Edinburgh Building, Cambridge CB2 8RU, UK

Published in the United States of America by Cambridge University Press, New York

www.cambridge.org
Information on this title: www.cambridge.org/9780521125857

First published 1989
This digitally printed version 2009

A catalogue record for this publication is available from the British Library

Library of Congress Cataloguing in Publication data

Gleason, John Joseph
Special education in context: an ethnographic study of
persons with developmental disabilities / John Joseph Gleason.
    p. cm.
Bibliography.
Includes index.
1. Developmentally disabled – Institutional care – United States –
Case studies.
2. Developmentally disabled – Education – United States – Case studies.
3. Special education – United States – Case studies.
I. Title.
HV1570.5.U65G58 1989
362.1'968 – dc19   88-37889CIP

ISBN 978-0-521-35187-4 Hardback
ISBN 978-0-521-12585-7 Paperback

To Patrick

Melinda,

I hope you journey through
doctoral studey is of
further spiritual awakening.

Good luck at the start

Contents

Figures and tables

Figures

Tables

Acknowledgments

The source material for this book comes from the residents of a state school for the mentally retarded. Each contributed in his or her own way. I am grateful for their participation. The staff of the school granted me access to the residents' lives. I hope this study will increase our understanding of persons with developmental disabilities.

The faculty at Harvard University influenced my development and the evolution of my inquiry. Dr Karen Watson-Gegeo cultivated my achievement by her own example as teacher, scholar, and researcher. Our conversations echo in the words of this book.

The administration of Rhode Island College and the faculty of the Department of Special Education provided me the opportunity for the development of this text. The editorial suggestions of the staff of Cambridge University Press enhanced the presentation of the content. The careful preparation of the manuscript is the work of Joyce Turner. Paul Weiner's illustrations were adapted by Jane Wilson.

This story is told as the result of a decade of personal sacrifice, financial support, and editorial assistance of my wife, Barrie. Words on a page cannot describe my love and appreciation. She touches every aspect of my life.

Introduction

It's not as bad as people say. They have a personality of their own. They'll try the patience of any newcomer. They really know newcomers by trying to watch them. Sometimes you see them with their arms around each other. You can write a book about what goes on here. *You* write about them because others are critical. They are not all that bad. (Nurse 1980)

This is a story over a five-year period about the residents of a state school for the mentally retarded, the severely and the profoundly mentally retarded and multiply handicapped.[1] I went as an anthropologist to the three apartments where they live, to observe the residents in their home. This study presents my observation of the residents as I observed them in the conduct of their daily life in the activity area of the apartments over two different periods.

Examples throughout the text from two periods of observation present a contrasting picture of life in the activity area of the apartments before and after the inauguration of federal legislation to provide individualized education programs for each of the 64 residents.[2]

Throughout the text the reader will encounter four different levels of analysis. The first level consists of raw data descriptions of the setting and of the residents. Descriptions are edited fieldnotes of the actual events, interactions, and observations made at the time. They are set off from the text to distinguish them from interpretations and theoretical explanations. Second are professional notes on residents and the setting, collected primarily from reports and resident records. Third are my interpretative statements about the residents and about professional statements. The interpretations develop into an explanation of the setting. Fourth are the theoretical statements that propose reconsideration of our understanding of residents and setting in social and cultural terms.

I set out to understand the residents from their own perspective through the evolution of a natural experiment in the setting between spring 1978 and spring 1982 and the analysis of three sets of data: observations of the residents in my fieldnotes, notes on the archive records of each resident, and historical information from documents, records, and books.

To ground my understanding and knowledge of the residents in

Table 1. *Chronology of the research program*

Phase 1	First period of research (January to June 1978) *Observation; Apartment M and apartment N: activity area* *Resident number: M = 29; N = 24*
	Quarantine of the institution (September 1979 to June 1980)
Phase 2	Second period of research (September 1979 to June 1980) *Observation; Apartment A: activity area and classrooms* *Resident number: A = 29 (15 from apartments M and N)*
	Application to review resident records (September 1980 to April 1981)
Phase 3	Third period of research (April to December 1981) *Record room of the institution*
Phase 4	Fourth period of research (April 1982 to April 1983) *Medical library of the institution*
Phase 5	Fifth period of research (January 1983 to August 1984) *Analysis, integration, explanation, and development of theory*

observation and explanation of their daily life on the ward, I conducted the research study in five phases. In phase 1, I sought to discover what the residents do on their own by observing social interaction on the ward. In phase 2, I compared and contrasted the residents' performance when professionals structure their activities with performance of residents on their own. In phase 3, I reviewed the residents' records. In phase 4, I examined historical reports, documents, and books to understand the research methods, models, and procedures historically used with the mentally retarded. Phase 5 began in January 1983 with the formal analysis, which included integration of all the data into an explanation and formulation of theory elaborated in this book. Table 1 outlines the research phases.

Early in 1978, I selected a state residential school for my field site. I was interested in the most severely handicapped individuals in an institution for two reasons. I was tired of debates on testing and the classification of handicaps into groups according to intelligence quotients and physiological characteristics. I was disillusioned with the curriculum programs in special education which placed such heavy emphasis on the individual attainment of a specific skill.

Nor was I enamored of the laws, recently passed, which mandated the assessment and prescription in a system of which I had become increasingly suspicious. With the laws, terminology had changed. "Mentally retarded" had become "developmentally disabled," but I was uncertain of the difference. The new handicap labels consisted of numerical listings found in the legislation. The procedures of practice, assessment, and programming were legislated. The new classifications created new divisions and categories. Upon state laws was superimposed federal law PL 94–142, Education of the Handicapped Act, which lent additional weight to state mandates but also introduced additional confusions to professionals trying to interpret guidelines and terminology. Educational discussions focused on compliance and rights. Absent from professional discussions in programs and public schools I visited were descriptions about what individuals did in the classrooms day-to-day, and discussion and examination of an individual's foibles and accomplishments. I decided the only way to understand what all this meant for the mentally retarded was to go and observe what the residents of the institution were doing and receiving as a result of the recent changes.

With over 15 years' professional experience in the field of special education, I knew that the complexity of their handicaps would test my knowledge (as they test any professional's knowledge). I knew also that the effect of the implementation of programs with this population would be most obvious because these individuals had not traditionally been the recipients of programs.

I entered the setting amidst the turmoil of an institution trying to cope with issues of mainstreaming, normalization, and deinstitutionalization. It was an institution in transition: an institution with a historical identity trying to establish a new identity while at the same time managing day-to-day life for over 1,200 residents. When I described what I was going to do, the most frequent refrain from the professionals was: "There is nothing going on there [in the apartment]. They don't do anything." When I told direct care staff in the apartment, however, they nodded or smiled with approval as if the idea had touched something about which they knew. The total number of residents observed in the apartments (A, M and N) in the two observation phases of the research was 67. I observed fifteen over the three years.

In Phase 1, I focused primarily on what the residents did on their own and secondarily on their participation in programmed lessons, conducted in the activity area common to apartments M and N. The activity area was the place to which they returned from other activities. Residents spent most of their time alone without staff, which allowed me the opportunity to witness firsthand what they did. Knowledge gained through the first period of observation was the basis for my subsequent understanding of the residents during the other phases. I realized I had come to learn about the residents in a way that differed substantially from the knowledge possessed by other staff members.

Right from the beginning, the ward arranged itself into a situation for a natural experiment. First, I was able to observe the residents on their own while they rested, or ate lunch or supper. These moments of anticipation of events, or reaction upon return to the apartment, were primary situations in which to observe transitions in their day. In the apartment I adjusted to the sights and sounds of the residents, attempting to interpret their movements, actions, giggles, gurgles, waves, and handshakes. I was interested in residents' response to the cycles of the day as well as to different individuals. I watched resident reaction to different members of the staff for contrasts and differences in the context of their interactions. I watched their responses and reactions to shifts of personnel at different times of the day.

In the first phase of the research, I watched interaction among residents. I was interested in the touching, holding, playing, or mirroring one another's rhythmic sounds in their vocalizations and movements. I watched and listened to the direct care staff. I was interested in their casual comments, which indicated how they interpreted a particular situation. For example, staff commenting on the same event used the labels "play" and "fight." I tried to understand the qualities of the interaction which provoked these different comments.

My data consisted of descriptions of what the residents did on their own and what they did in their interactions with direct care staff and professional staff. Professionals were informal with their greetings, hand-shakes, and waves when passing through the ward or visiting spontane-ously with a resident. They were formal in the conduct of their care and treatment of the residents. In phase 1, clues to staff understanding of an event were additional stepping stones towards understanding the residents.

Implementation of the mandated programs during the school year 1978–79 was the first full year during which programming was attempted for all residents. My study was interrupted at this time when a quarantine restricted access to the building for all but essential personnel. Total programming for all residents was achieved during 1979–80, overlapping the second period of observation. Subsequently programs for each resident were updated in the annual review when performance reflected progress on individual objectives. Activities of daily living such as feeding, dressing, brushing teeth, and showering were reinforced by teaching developmental skills in individual, group, and class sessions. Resident life became structured into an escalating series of skills, abilities, objectives, and priorities set by the professional staff.

The implementation of programming for the residents upon my return to the setting for the second period of observation (1979–80) was in sharp contrast to the previous period (Phase 1) in which the resident programs were limited to positioning in the activity area and the conduct of basic

4

care and activities of daily living. Phase 2 of the research with the residents involved observation of programmed activities on a different floor and apartment. I observed resident participation with staff in these activities.

Both in the classroom and on the ward, resident life was programmed to teach developmental skills such as feeding, social interaction, and communication. Teachers assessed achievement according to the criteria of specific objectives. Apartment A residents were in classrooms and therapy sessions morning and afternoon. Their entire day was scheduled and managed. The only exception was the rest period between sessions.

With the change to total programming, the residents were now involved in lessons and therapy designed to teach, train and develop, and manage their behavior. Thus in phase 2 I could compare their behavior and performance in the structured and programmed activities conducted by the professionals with their behavior in phase 1 during the rest period, when they were left on their own. The 15 residents observed during both phases provided the basis for this comparison across the three years.

During phase 2 I systematically collected data on the residents' social behavior in different contexts: the apartment activity area, the classroom lessons, and socialization class. Seeing the differences, difficulties, and frustrations that staff encountered in getting the residents to conform to the criteria of an objective in a lesson, I came to understand differences in interpretation of the residents' behavior.

Before the advent of total programming, I realized that I possessed data on what the residents were able to do. I had comparative data in my fieldnotes. First, I could compare and contrast the type and the quality of the residents' interaction with one another during the rest period (1) in the combined activity area with 53 other residents in 1978 with (2) Apartment A's activity area holding only 29 residents, from 1979 to 1980. Secondly, having anticipated the advent of total programming, I wanted to see if the residents behaved differently during the rest period after they had participated in structured programs throughout the day. During phase 2, the teachers had initiated a socialization class in which residents from three classrooms participated in teacher-directed social activities to promote peer interactions. I was interested in learning what the teachers knew about the residents' peer interaction. What type of socialization program would they design to promote interaction among the residents? How would the residents respond to such directed socialization? Since the socialization class followed right after the rest period, I could follow the residents into the socialization class after observing them on their own. I could observe any variation and differences in their behavior in the two contexts. I could compare and contrast the social behavior of the residents as it evolved in their daily circumstances with their demonstrated ability in a programmed activity constructed to teach social behavior. I could compare and contrast the qualities of the interaction, the length of time of the activity, and the structural characteristics of the lesson.

The reorganization provided a different set of circumstances in the two phases of observation. I could compare and contrast the residents' behavior given a minimum of activity and programs (phase 1) with greater intervention and involvement by the professional staff a year later (phase 2).

I left the ward in June 1980 when I was confident that my interpretations of the meaning in the residents' behavior had significance. To fill in the data in my fieldnotes, in April 1981 I began the formal investigation of the archive records on each of the 64 residents I had observed in apartments M, N, and A.

In phase 3 of the research, the resident records enriched my own data in the fieldnotes. The resident records broadened the institutional picture of the residents in references found in evaluations, programs, and objectives. What the residents were expected to do and what they did in fact achieve through the programs is documented. The records provided a description of the setting, further documenting what was going on within the institution, the buildings, and wards throughout the various states of transition and across the two periods of observation. A picture of the institution and the residents emerged from the two sources of data, the fieldnotes, and the residents' records. The resident's record, consisting of up to five folders, contained 300–1,000 pages of accumulated reports and notes on each individual. The reports included initial impressions upon admission, daily progress notes, referrals to other departments or institutions, accident and injury reports, restraining records, and clinical evaluations. The reports detailed an individual's personal history prior to and throughout his or her institutional life. The picture is a detailed analysis of the steps taken by the family and staff at the institution to provide care and treatment for the resident. The reports document the developing awareness of the complexity of handicaps from a variety of perspectives: medical, psychological, therapeutic, social, and educational.

I investigated the records on each individual for statements which indicated what the reporter knew about what the resident did on his own. I was interested in statements about their expression, or about meaning attributed to their behavior. I looked for descriptions of what the residents did with one another, how they interacted with those with whom they lived. Finally, I was interested in "off-the-cuff" comments made by the staff about the residents, remarks about what they did which indicated their identification of characteristics, traits, features of their personality which the staff characterized as typical, or as unique to the individual. I wanted to find out how the staff saw the residents, and how they commented on them over and above the objective and standardized clinical language.

Introduction

I was interested in the identification and documentation of purposeful action by the residents. Did the professionals or the attendants identify what the residents did on their own? The extent to which the residents were thought to demonstrate purposeful interaction seemed to be an important first step in planning lessons or activities. The records held the key to determine what the professional staff knew about residents.

The clinical interpretations informed me of additional problems, impediments, and handicaps that influenced the resident's life; I marveled at their ability despite the burden of their handicap. Moreover, I realized that the information, although painfully thorough and comprehensive, was descriptive not of the individual but of his handicap. The programming consisted of efforts to ameliorate the handicapping condition. It began with the handicap, and the description of all possible combinations of handicaps, and proceeded with the aim of improving the functioning of the individual with the handicap.

To set the study in historical context, I returned to the institution for phase 4 of the research. Looking for consistency in the way mental retardation was regarded, I reviewed the historical records at the institution to trace the continuity in the application of the clinical experimental framework. The historical bifurcation of the normal and the pathological provided an interpretive model for understanding the origin of many of the present complications in understanding the residents and in practice.

Briefly, I documented the fact that the severely and profoundly mentally retarded and multiply handicapped, previously the custodial mentally retarded, were considered separate from the other residents of the institution. They received only custodial care. This state of benign neglect persisted until present-day involvement and intervention following the passage of PL 94–142 (1975). This federal legislation mandated the development of individualized educational programs in the least restrictive environment for each person with developmental disabilities. The severely and profoundly mentally retarded and multiply handicapped were from the beginning of custodial care the subject of clinical classification. For example, Howe's (1847) categorization in his field study determined the condition of the "idiots" in the Commonwealth of Massachusetts. Simultaneously I traced – through the writings of the founding fathers – the origins of special education services and programs, programs for the mentally retarded, and the development of clinical examination and research, to show the continuity of clinical descriptions and practice as the primary basis of our knowledge of the mentally retarded.

During analysis of my fieldnotes in phase 5, I realized that many of my fieldnotes described the structure and organization of the apartment of professional practice rather than the residents themselves. This was not

7

my intended focus, but nevertheless it was indicative of the pervasiveness of structured programs during this period of research. Sometimes, focus on the lesson or program nearly consumed my entire description. This precipitated a confrontation with my own professional knowledge in special education. Would I continue to focus on the lessons as the key, and base my understanding on what the professionals were doing, and thus concentrate on institutional processes? Or would I commit myself to a comprehensive understanding of the residents? This was my struggle throughout the analysis of the fieldnotes and development of a theory of the setting. I needed to *forgo* my professional knowledge and attachments to focus on the residents.

I had to relearn what I had learned during phase 1 – continually readjusting my expectations to the reality of what the residents did, in all its subtlety. Only by paying attention to the residents could I begin to make statements about the efficacy of structured programmed activities, not only in terms of the characteristics of the residents' interaction in the classrooms with teachers but also in terms of their interaction with one another in the apartment.

I applied formal analysis to my fieldnotes throughout the course of my reflection and preparation for the writing of this description. By formal analysis, I mean the review, study, and the decision to adopt an interpretation for specific selected events in the data.

Although I was separating and categorizing data, I could also reintegrate the information once I had pulled it apart. This method of reduction and reintegration allowed me to compare events and behaviors for residents and staff over the three years. The research questions which evolved in the course of the analysis and guided the description of the setting were the following: (1) What are the patterns of behavior of the residents in the conduct of everyday life? And what are their patterns when left on their own? (2) What do the residents do in the apartment activity area on their own and in structured program activities? (3) What patterns do staff become aware of in their day-to-day care? (4) What are the characteristics of the individual labeled severely and profoundly mentally retarded and multiply handicapped? These questions were subsumed under one general research question: what do the individuals called residents, and clinically labeled severely and profoundly mentally retarded and multiply handicapped, *do* in the conduct of everyday life on the ward in a state school for the mentally retarded?

To answer these questions I had in mind a detailed description found in Itard's *The Wild Boy of Aveyron* and Itard's attempts to educate Victor (1801–6). This classic report provides a description of Victor's capabilities, but also of the statements and objectives of the teacher, Itard. From observations of the residents on their own I had knowledge of their capabilities outside educational and therapeutic programs. I was interested in describing their performance on objectives in interactions with teachers. The challenge was to discover the qualities and characteristics of their communication and interaction in both contexts, in order to understand better the complexities of their multiple disabilities and the influence of those disabilities on functioning.

Each chapter of this book begins with an introduction to the historical context of the principal ideas advanced in the chapter (Scheerenberger 1983). While not an exhaustive study of special education, each introduction highlights the recurrent themes in special education, from the founding personalities in the development of special education to the care and treatment specifically of the severely and profoundly mentally retarded and multiply handicapped.

Chapter 1 introduces the residents, the setting, and the program. The description of the setting introduces social, political, legal, and cultural influences which presently guide practice. The residents are introduced through a description of initial impressions on an introductory tour of the building and the apartments in which lived the most severely handicapped individuals. Finally, the program is described in terms of the formal processes by which knowledge about the residents is communicated among the direct care staff and other professionals. Chapter 1 includes a description of the systems for collecting information for the case record, and a summary clinical statement that describes the residents.

Chapter 2 guides the reader through a change in perspective: from understanding the clinical configuration of an individual with the label "severe and profound mental retardation and multiple handicaps" to understanding the individual in his or her own terms by adopting his or her perspective.

Chapter 3 presents an example of the spontaneous interaction between two individuals, Danial and Thomas, to illustrate the change in the definition of their ability. This interaction challenges the definition of their ability strictly in terms of mental, social, and behavioral characteristics, stages, and skills.

While chapter 3 describes what Danial and Thomas do on their own, chapter 4 describes their interaction with staff, including direct care staff, professionals and volunteers, and the friction in the interaction between residents and staff. The significance of the contrast in performance reveals itself to be the restricted interpretation by staff of resident performance within the objectives and behavioral criteria of the lesson and the therapeutic activities, the focused interpretation and evaluation of the individuals' performance in terms of skill and abilities, and implicit and explicit judgements in terms of personal conventions and norms for participation. The friction comes from these assumptions, standards, expectations, and conventions, rather than from the difficulties that result from the handicap.

The residents, a remarkably heterogeneous and complex group of individuals, have evolved specific patterns of interaction and communication which are learned and shared. In the implementation of educational and therapeutic lessons, they are exposed systematically to a structured approach to their diversity. Chapter 5 explores the fundamental tension which arises when our programs are aligned to be consistent with the residents' ability, and connected to their experience. In essence, this requires the acknowledgement that their variation and difference (especially demonstrated by the severely and profoundly mentally retarded and multiply handicapped in this setting) has its own merits. Clinical characteristics and conditions give only limited definition of their experience and ability, and define only generally their relationship to one another. This explanation rests on a redefinition of *normal* rather than on attempts to normalize these individual differences.

The definition of the individual's potential can be found in the purposeful actions and behaviors which they demonstrate in their everyday life. If we aim to ground our practice in an essential understanding of their human differences, of the dynamics of their performance within interactions, and of the meaning constructed in their participation, we must realign our definitions of "normal," "appropriate," and "potential" in terms of what it means *to them*. Our concepts of life, and of the quality of *their* life, are enhanced through the understanding of what they do.

Notes

1 The names of all residents have been changed to preserve anonymity. Staff are identified only by the professional discipline that describes their function and role. The terms used in reference to the residents are those of the staff.
2 The total number of residents in apartments M, N, and A is 67. In the text, 64 is the number of residents who were present in the activity area throughout the greater part of the study.

I

An institution in transition

The historical context

Since the 1800s, mentally retarded individuals have been understood primarily through descriptions of their *condition*. Attempts at diagnosis, treatment, and cure of that condition take precedence over the study of the person in a social context. Several elements influence these attempts: (1) Establishment of a precise demarcation between normal and abnormal. Medicine, psychology, physical anthropology, and education seek to objectify this division and the range of variation and differences in the human species. (2) The biological basis of the condition as the root of clinical study. Determination of the cause of mental retardation is sought with the aim of eventual elimination and eradication of the condition. (3) Education and training of the individual to acquire socially, culturally and developmentally appropriate skills. Intervention is based on development of norms, criteria and levels demonstrating more normal status. (4) Compassion for the profound nature of handicaps. Historically this concern increasingly becomes justification for what is done to the severely and profoundly mentally retarded and multiply handicapped in the name of compassion, philanthropy, goodwill, and a developing social conscience.

The history of special education is in part a history of individuals who took an active interest in the mentally retarded and multiply handicapped. In all the historical documentation of the educational classics, the reports of superintendents, the case studies, and the historic literature, who is the subject and the object of practice?

Philippe Pinel (1745–1826), the founder of modern psychiatry, applied to idiots the positivism of ideas in the sciences and the medical model of nineteenth-century Paris. He was the first to render a clinical distinction of mental functions of the same kind that was applied to bodily functions. He was the first to develop descriptions of mental characteristics into a typology of mental disease (Foucault, 1976).

Pinel offered a clinical description of idiotism as the fifth species of mental derangement after melancholia, mania without delirium, mania with delirium, and dementia.[1] His pioneering attempts to distinguish idiots from indigents, vagabonds, criminals, the insane, deranged, demented, alienated, or extravagant, and his historic unchaining of the inmates at the asylum Hôpital Bicêtre (1794) earned him the title of savior of the mentally ill. Although Pinel separated idiots from sufferers from other identified mental illnesses, he offered limited hope for their improvement. The undifferentiated nature of idiocy and the pervasiveness of its effect on the individual led Pinel to the conclusion that the only treatment was unchained custodial care. The conviction in Pinel's conclusions represented nineteenth-century positivism in medical scientific thought on idiots.

In 1800, Pinel clinically observed and assessed a feral child, the Wild Boy of Aveyron:

We know the other details of his life from the time he entered society, his judgement always limited to the objects of basic needs; his attention captured slowly by the sight of food, or by means of living independently, a strongly acquired habit; the total absence of subsequent development of his intellectual faculties with regard to every other object. *Do these assert that the child ought to be characterized among the children suffering from idiocy and insanity, and that there is no hope whatever of obtaining some measure of success through systematic and continued instruction?* (Lane, 1979: 69; emphasis added)

I will examine the truths that follow and will indicate if the so called wild boy of Aveyron can be submitted with well founded instruction and *acculturation* or if it is necessary to abandon this agreeable prospect and confine him simply in our asylums with other unfortunate victims of an incomplete and damaged constitution. (Lane, 1979: 64; emphasis added)

After detailed examination of the behavior of the Wild Boy, which he compared with that of normal children and of other idiots within the asylum, Pinel disallowed the likelihood of acculturation and, based on the diagnosis of idiocy, made a prognosis of "incurable."

Jean-Marc-Gaspard Itard (1774–1838) became known as the father of special education for applying his medical training and clinical skills of observation beyond diagnosis to the education and care of the Wild Boy. Taking up the care of the feral animal-man he called Victor (1801–6), Itard sought to discover his capabilities. Itard's historic challenge to Pinel's diagnosis of idiocy inaugurated clinical observation and analysis of behavior and training of the senses (Boyd, 1914:10). Referring to Pinel's identification of Victor as an idiot, Itard stated:

This identity led to the inevitable conclusion that, attacked by a malady hitherto regarded as *incurable*, he [Victor] was not capable of any kind of sociability or instruction.

I never shared this unfavorable opinion and in spite of the truth of the picture and the justice of the parallels I dared to conceive certain hopes. I founded them on my part upon the double consideration of the cause and the curability of this apparent idiocy. (Itard, 1962:6–7; emphasis added)

Itard based his clinical observation and analysis of Victor on the improvement and development of the intellect by the isolation and the separate stimulation of each of the senses (Boyd, 1914:73). He stated his pedagogical aims: "I classified under five principal aims the mental and moral education of the Wild Boy of Aveyron" (Itard, 1962:10–11).

Through instructional tasks and activities, Itard bombarded the boy's senses and nurtured the development of speech in the context of everyday life. Itard linked the introduction of speech to the satisfaction of physical desires and needs, such as a request for milk, even though Victor's repeated attempts at speech were frustrating and later abandoned. The presence or absence of speech was seen then as the distinguishing characteristic along the man-animal/man-idiot continuum.

Attempting to restore Victor to normality, Itard promoted gradual enticement to the comforts of social and cultural life. He tried to educate the animal-man to function as man within society by awakening the natural human sensitivities of the emotions and speech from the dormant facilities of Victor's organs. His affiliation to society was linked to the gradual attachment to functioning within society.

If Victor were unable to acquire this affiliation, Itard would have to accept Pinel's diagnosis of idiocy and abandon Victor as an idiot to the asylum – the place where idiots lived out an existence by the benevolence of the state. Itard did not think that Victor in his present state as an idiot could assimilate into society.

Itard changed the substance and the focus of the clinical scrutiny of medicine from a search for the underlying pathology of idiocy (begun by Pinel) to a clinical scrutiny of individual psychology and educational potential. In this way, Itard's experiment with Victor's acculturation encompassed a new application of the scientific skills of clinical observation to individual psychological and mental states, as well as to characteristics of behavior, and a test of the philosophy of education of the individual.

With the knowledge obtained from the observation of Victor's free and spontaneous exploration of the environment, Itard also attempted cultivation of the senses through social intercourse. Itard isolated each of the senses, targeting them at particular times in the course of instruction. Instruction proceeded by exercises to improve separately each of the sense organs (Boyd, 1914:73). Introducing Victor to social and cultural conventions and training his mental faculties were treated separately. Itard's case study, *The Wild Boy of Aveyron* (1962), was a record of the application of the clinical method of observation, and of the sequence of interaction and instruction in the educational process.

The aims of the educational program were to be achieved through the following pedagogical steps: (1) clinical observation, to understand as thoroughly as possible the specific characteristics of Victor's nature; (2) planned presentation of educational tasks and sequences of instruction to develop Victor's unique characteristics; (3) a calculated method of interacting with Victor to manage his behavior into socially acceptable patterns.

The educational experiment which Itard undertook turned out to be more a test of the likelihood of acculturation than a study of the origin and nature of idiocy. The Paris Academy of Science reminded a disappointed Itard of the criteria by which his experiment should be judged: "the pupil ought to be compared *only to himself*" (Séguin, 1907:21. Emphasis added). Itard's frustration evolved because he felt that no progress was being achieved in his struggle "against the obstinacy of the organ." Victor learned what was expected of him to survive: to get food and to avoid punishment or reprisal from Itard, such as the withholding of food. Itard's attention to the task, the experiment, and the analytical ways in which he conducted the instruction, focused his evaluation on achievement of educational aims. What Victor actually learned is not known and may in fact still lie between the lines of the text of *The Wild Boy of Aveyron*. The ways in which Victor learned and adjusted to the characteristics of Itard, the subtle manipulation of the tasks to thwart Itard, and the ways in which Victor used his understanding of the situation and the context to protect himself in this environment have not been told. The instruction described in Itard's book was linear, directed at the achievement of an educational goal through the bombarding of specific senses. He pursued this course until failure was acknowledged or he became frustrated, in which case he selected another educational aim and another approach.

The medical-clinical educational experiment and analysis was revolutionary for the time. In fact, this case study serves as a model for educational initiatives with the handicapped to this day. But there were limits to Itard's vision of Victor. This case study reflects Itard's aims and goals. Systematic instruction focused on circumscribed areas and did not consider critical relationships among the human systems and within the context of teaching and learning situations.

The basic assumptions for the education of the mentally retarded which develop out of this account include: (1) clinical diagnosis and assessment of physiological and mental condition; (2) determination of characteristics of idiocy as a condition which distinguishes the individual from other members of the society and culture; (3) stimulation of innate but dormant qualities in the imperfect organ of the mind; (4) activation of the mind through stimulation of the senses; (5) complete analysis of the condition and provision of adequate educational material and programs; and (6) inculcation of culturally appropriate behaviors.

Edouard Séguin (1812–80), a student of Itard, applied his clinical and analytical skills to distinguish between physiological and neurological characteristics and the various levels of functional behavior he observed within the general class of the feebleminded. Séguin, often referred to as the "apostle of the idiots," refined the analytical observation applied by Itard in the education of Victor. He expanded and systematized Itard's five educational aims into a method to train the organs. For Séguin, idiocy was a sub-category of feeblemindedness. Séguin's preference was to work with those individuals at the lower end of the spectrum of functional ability.

The aim of Séguin's physiological education was to free the mind from the defect of the organs. By examination and analysis of neurological structures and bodily functions, he attempted to direct treatment towards the underlying neurological structures. The method consisted of medical observation and analysis of the whole individual: first, the organic faculties, the functions of the cerebral, muscular, and sensory system; and secondly, the training of the senses and the organs as a vehicle to thought and development.

For 18 months, Séguin undertook the education of an idiot boy by his method. Within this time he was able to teach him to remember, to compare, and to speak, write, and count. After the success of this singular case brought him acclaim, he opened a school and applied his method to ten pupils. The Parisian Academy of Science declared that Séguin had *solved* the problem of the education of idiots (Boyd, 1914:92).

The combination of clinical examination of the whole individual, the observation and analysis of functional behavior, the attention to neurological signs and characteristics, and the distinction between different types of idiot based on these functional behaviors and neurological signs were all significant. With Séguin the clinical method became an analytical tool to help distinguish the various traits, characteristics, and symptoms of idiots. More importantly, the clinical method was applied to instruction, in the form of analysis of a specific ability and the design of an instructional device to develop that ability.

Séguin's contribution was twofold. First, he developed clinical categories within the general classification of feeblemindedness. To distinguish between the different types of feeblemindedness was to determine the application of the method of instruction. Not only were physiological signs and characteristics important, but also manifestations of certain behavioral traits. He drew the relationship between functional behavior and specific organs. Through examination and listing of these traits, he developed a typology of clinical categories and behavioral manifestation.

The typologies of idiocy were to change, and as knowledge accrued and the distinction between characteristics and behaviors evolved, the first physiological *and* behavioral descriptions took root with the work of Séguin (1880). Séguin's second contribution was to incorporate the clinical method into educational pedagogy. Underlying this method was the assumption of a correspondence between the *organ*, the functional *behavior* which was traced to that organ, and the ability of the instructional procedure and *device* to train the organ, thereby influencing the functional behavior.

Samuel Gridley Howe (1801–76), founder of the first publicly supported school for idiots and feebleminded in the United States, was prompted by observation of the successful treatment in 1839 of an idiotic, blind, non ambulatory, paralytic child. Aware of Séguin's physiological method, Howe enlisted his aid in the design of the instructional program. R. A. Richards, Howe's first teacher at the Massachusetts School for the Feebleminded, was sent to France to learn Séguin's method. Séguin's instructional program remained essentially intact throughout Howe's tenure, and was the basis of instructional programs under Dr. Walter E. Fernald.

In 1894 Fernald reported to the Association of Medical Officers of American Institutions for Idiotic and Feebleminded Persons on the methods employed in the care and training of lower-grade custodial cases. In one of the rare descriptions of this class of feebleminded living within the custodial department of the institutions, Fernald stated:

These children are often feeble physically, perhaps incapable of walking without assistance, of feeding or dressing themselves or of making their bodily wants known. Some of them are utterly stupid and listless. Others are very restless and excitable, with marked mischievous and destructive tendencies, such as moving and destroying clothing, breaking window glass, table crockery and furniture. Many cases have very untidy and disgusting personal habits. (Fernald, 1896:24)

As Superintendent of the Massachusetts School for the Feebleminded, Fernald admitted several hundred "low-grade custodial cases."

When admitted nearly every one of these children was noisy, untidy, stubborn and intractable generally. Few of them had been under any sort of control or discipline. One had not been out of doors in three years. Several had been confined in barred rooms at home. How to care for them was a discouraging problem. The wards were veritable bedlams. The children shrieked and made dreadful noises, tore off and destroyed their clothing and seemed utterly unmanageable. Their attendants were appalled and discouraged at the apparent hopelessness of trying to bring any degree of order out of such chaos, and were almost ready to resign in a body. (Fernald, 1896:24)

The practical prescription offered within his report for the attendants included: (1) frequent changes of personal clothing after baths and toileting to decrease "the characteristic disagreeable odor" they emit; (2) generous allotment of nutritious food accompanied by sufficient allotment of *time* to eat the food; (3) administration of abundant amounts of water despite efforts to restrict intake so as to keep them from wetting the bed; (4) excursions into the open air and exercise throughout the year; (5) the availability of numerous playthings (Fernald, 1896:25).

Fernald's first concern was the *basic adjustment of care to the particular needs of the groups of individuals within the institution.* Ordering the chaos began not by lessening the work for the attendants but by providing careful arrangement of schedules to promote proper eating habits, increase the frequency of activities, provide basic health care, introduce new toys to their environment, and allow the exploration of the environment outside the asylum building whatever the New England season. The principles which Fernald advocated to guide practice are preventative: adjustment to the needs of the individual, including the subtle recognition of the *time* differences which exist in the conduct of their everyday activities and promotion of continuous experience within the environment.

The attendants in this description provided the order within the dormitories of the asylum; but education rested within the patient, persistent teacher.

Right here I want to emphasize my firm conviction that it is utter nonsense to attempt this training of low-grade cases unless it is done in the most painstaking, conscientious and thorough manner by a teacher who thoroughly believes in the real value of this work. (Fernald, 1896:30)

Teachers with such conviction were sought to provide a type of education or training to the individual within the custodial department. "Indeed, books, slates and the conventional curriculum of the school-room are not for these low-grade children. Yet all of this training is education in the truest sense" (Fernald, 1896: 31).

The principles upon which the habit training of low-grade custodial cases was based were rooted in the observable conditions of the difference, the absence or loss of ability, deficit and deficiency. Education in such cases became the exercise of mind over matter – the will of the teacher over the matter of the custodial low grades. To overcome the presumed absence of volition, teacher conviction and habit training were substituted.

One of the most troublesome features in the care of these low-grade cases is the frequency of untidy personal habits ... In many cases the indolence of the child is a potent factor. We must cause the child to lose the habit of being untidy and to acquire the habit of being clean and decent. The general raising of the physiological standard, both mentally and physically, which results from the regulation of diet, the careful bathing, the out-door exercise and the physical and other training, often correct the untidy habits without special treatment. (Fernald, 1896:26)

Fernald recognized characteristics of differences between low-grade custodial cases which distinguished them from normal children. This recognition justified differential treatment. The need for the total awakening and development of the individual was made necessary by the profound nature of their handicap and the resulting cycle of a sedentary life.

The legislative act of 1886 (Commonwealth of Massachusetts, 1886 Chap. 298) provided a charter statement of the principal divisions around which the formal structure of the Massachusetts School for the Feebleminded was organized: custodial and school. The act codified the right of the overseers of the institution to make discretionary judgements about the potential of the individual and the benefits to be derived from placement in either department upon admission and from attendance at the school.

Individuals placed within the custodial department were recognized as belonging to a different grade or kind of feeblemindedness. Their segregation within an asylum building isolated geographically from the other residents and buildings was another indicator of their differential treatment. One assumed difference was the absence of will which could only be activated by training. Intense training of the senses was to develop the will to explore the environment and to progress through the acquisition of skills and the performance of conventional behaviors. Progress was marked by the development of volition, when the individual began to exercise control over behavior and to develop intellectual faculties. Advancement within the institution was marked by transfer from the custodial department to the school.

This transfer entailed the demonstration to the trustees of the institution, the caretakers, teachers, and the medical staff, of the expected skills and behaviors. For the custodial low grade, this assumed active participation in the training program, the learning and incorporation into their behavioral repertoire of new skills, and the ability to participate successfully in interactions with their caretakers. The criteria applied to their performance was the ability to acquire expected learning patterns and to participate in socially appropriate ways. The comparisons applied to custodial low grades were normal childhood and infancy patterns. The assumption that these comparisons were appropriate influenced the development of education and training of the custodial individuals until the present.

Summary

Instruction and programming in the twentieth century have been based on Séguin's methods. Clinical examination of the individual determined type and level of idiocy, and from that description a treatment, an instructional device, or a program of activities was prescribed.

Thus an individual was known by his classification as an idiot. The success of the method in one particular case was generalized to a class of individuals and then adopted as an instructional system. This cycle repeated itself throughout the history of special education. Séguin's medical-clinical analysis was central to the design and organization of instructional tasks. Séguin formalized into a model what Pinel initiated in his separation of the idiots into a unique class and in his formulation of a descriptive definition, and what Itard initiated as the application of clinical analysis to instruction in an educational experiment.

The institution

The state school for the mentally retarded in which this study takes place is an institution in transition. We shall consider what effect a combination of changes in the internal organization of the institution and in the physical plant had on the setting and the residents. Changes in the administrative organization, the implementation of a developmentally oriented skills program for individual residents, and the renovation of existing facilities produced day-to-day crises which confused and frustrated all personnel trying to implement and change programs simultaneously. This kaleidoscope of influences on the setting had one common rationale: the aim of better serving the residents.

Ostensibly, the goal of the changes was the enhancement of quality of life for residents living within the institution, by means of normalizing the institution to meet the residents' individual needs in an environment as close to mainstream cultural standards as possible. Wards became apartments; shower stalls replaced group showers and the shower slab; dormitory living space became individual and semi-private rooms; large cafeteria and feeding areas on the ward were replaced with small, home-like dining areas. Mainstreaming implied culturally standardized norms of behavior. For a resident, this implied movement when possible out of the institution into the community (deinstitutionalization) to a less restrictive environment or community residence, for example a group home or sheltered workshop environment, or a community residence.

For 15 years prior to my arrival, the institution had developed a reorganization and implementation plan. For the institution to receive Title XIX funds (1975–77) and to comply with federal and state mandated guidelines, it had to provide individualized educational programs within the least restrictive environment for each of the residents. Title XIX funds were federally appropriated to improve personnel, services, and programs for residents in state hospitals and schools. To receive funds, schools performed assessments on residents as the basis for developing programs and securing staff and services. The assessment for the Title XIX funds was the initial assessment and one which formed the basis for the individualized programs for the residents under subsequent federal and state laws. With the mandates of federal and state laws, additional assessments and specific educational plans were developed and reviewed annually. The annual reviews of the individualized educational programs reflected the organizational plan for improved functioning described in the institution's curriculum of skills sequences. The individualized program for the residents outlined a progression from assessed functional level, for example sensory stimulation, to the highest level of skill development. Individual educational plans complemented the reorganization of the institution.

At this time (1974), the state schools were subject to class action suits and a consent decree to secure for all class members (the residents) the right to care and treatment that met minimal constitutional requirements. Under the U.S. District Court for the state, the judge (through a court monitor) established a framework for providing suitable living environments and rehabilitation services. The court monitor had an immediate influence on the appointment of professional staff and inauguration of resident programs. In addition, the school had undertaken a multi-million dollar renovation project. The new federal Secretary of Health and Human Services threatened to stop funding for construction projects, licensing, and the appropriation of other funds for the continuation of the existing services and renovations if the state did not match the federal funds. These funds were necessary for the institution to overcome the deficiencies noted in state and federal inspections and audits.

In this highly political and legally complex atmosphere, with two changes in state government and two different superintendents at the school and with an influx of new professionals under several service contracts, I conducted my observations on the ward now referred to as an apartment.

The setting

The large state school for the mentally retarded had functioned formerly as a self-contained institution providing total care for its residents. Built at the turn of the century, its architectural style and the conditions of the buildings themselves suggest another era in the care and treatment of the

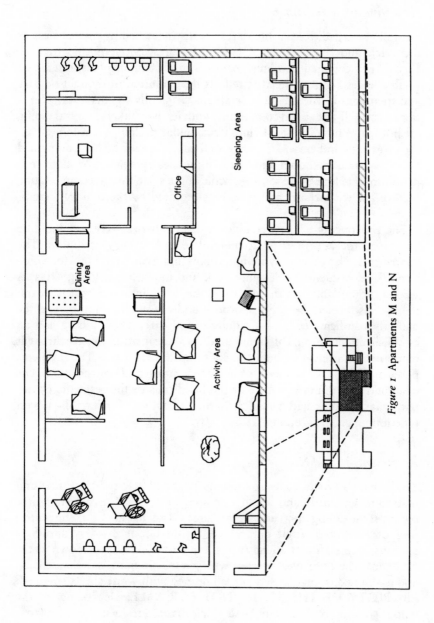

Figure 1 Apartments M and N

mentally retarded. Recent buildings are distinguished by the newness of the brick and the absence of Gothic features. Modern construction, clusters of octagonal buildings made up of little apartments, resembled small villages. The architecture reflects the evolution of thought on care and treatment of the mentally retarded. Originally the institution functioned as a self-contained community, with its own bakery, central dining facilities, and buildings for living. Rectangular buildings accommodated the growing numbers of custodial total care clients which accompanied the post-war baby boom and German measles epidemics. Modern residences imitate home-like settings, while at the same time accommodating the host of wheelchairs and stretchers required by the multiply handicapped.

The apartments where I conducted this fieldwork were in a building built three decades ago to accommodate a different population. The apartments, classrooms, swimming pool, and gym were built for vocational level residents to develop work and independent living skills. A second population has found its home here in more recent years: individuals labeled "severely and profoundly mentally retarded and the multiply handicapped," who required total care. The building had an established reputation. Different buildings in the institution have different reputations, in terms of both the staff and the residents. The problems posed by both are the target of endless scrutiny and conversation. The profound and multiple nature of the handicaps of the residents of this particular building had gained them the reputation of being "the lowest functioning on the grounds."

Apartments M and N

The activity area shared by apartments M and N held residents' toys and mats, dining utensils, and adaptive equipment (fig. 1). The room has three sections: the dining, mat, and storage areas. The mat area was the central part of the room, itself partitioned by three-foot dividers into four sections. The staff could lean over these partitions to peer down at the residents. The floor was covered with gymnastic mats, sandbag chairs, and cushioned triangular wedges, all draped with white sheets stamped: PROPERTY OF THE STATE, NOT FOR SALE. Depending on the amount of sand contained in the sandbag chairs, a resident could look out over the other residents but no one seemed able to move arm or leg once placed in it. Contact with the other residents was virtually impossible from this position. Here, residents scheduled for the "positioning program" on these various cushioned devices spent most of their day.

On the first day of my observations, I walked through the activity area. Prominent against the white sheets and nestled everywhere throughout the activity area were a few toys: a pale yellow duck with paint scraped from fingernail scratches, its orange beak now white because it was sucked upon so often; a wooden boat with wheels, its side chipped; a turquoise ball held by Kenneth; a white and red Fisher-Price lawn mower with colored balls inside the top dome lying by Danial. A football sat on its own mat; blocks and foam rubber balls resembled basketballs in miniature. A doll with disheveled hair and upturned arms pulled in different directions was placed beside selected residents. A puppet head of Goofey and Micky Mouse sat beside the silver plastic guns. Other objects were overhead. Hung from strings were little dolls and a ring donut that danced in the air when hit by attendants passing by. Plastic mosaic clowns stood midway up the wall around the room. Interspersed with the clowns were toy animal characters in wooden frames smiling over the whole scene. Except for the seasonal changes, this was the extent of the permanent decoration.

Attendants sat on stainless steel chairs while supervising the residents. One rocking chair belonged to Benjamin. The first year of the study, Benjamin sat in the far end of the room and rocked in his chair, one foot tucked under the thigh of the other. He pressed his foot to the floor to rock the chair back and forth. The first year the teachers brought a table into the activity area for educational activities. Joseph sat in front of a colored blue box with holes of different shapes, to be filled with a yellow moon, a red cross, a blue square, or a green star. With or without Joseph, the shapes sat on the table.

A standing locker, a clothes bin and rows of wheelchairs and bed stretchers were the only other objects to be found in the activity area. The only change in these objects each week was in the arrangement of the wheelchairs and bed stretchers. Seasonal changes in decorations provided relief from the sameness in the environment throughout the two periods of observation. Traditional decorations marked the introduction and passing of each of the holidays. The seasons of the decorations often overlapped. In March, an aluminum Christmas tree on one wall marked the December holiday while the green shamrocks and leprechauns on the office window facing the activity area signaled the coming holiday. With the passing of St. Patrick's Day, the aluminum Christmas tree and the shamrocks were removed. Easter rabbits appeared right after the shamrocks, with elaborately colored eggs and baby chicks as a collage on the office window.

At mealtime, staff moved residents from mats and chairs and stretchers to a corner of the room which served as the dining area. In this section was a long folding table piled with bowls and dishes and specially designed spoons to feed the residents. Into this area, the meal cart rolled from the kitchen preparation area diagonally across the hall.

A second room of the apartment was a bedroom, a maze of thirty crib-style beds separated by metal cabinets. Each hospital-type bed with collapsible sides was covered with a brightly colored bedspread. When all the beds were made at the end of the feeding time, the room was a bright collection of blues, reds and yellows. The variety of colors contrasted with army-green lockers with an occasional name or photo taped to it. On the bed or in the cabinet were personal clothes or special toys.

Intersecting both rooms was a glassed-in office from which staff observed the 25 or so residents who lived there at any one time (or, in the activity area of the apartments during the first period of the research, 40 to 50 residents positioned there for most of the day). Behind the office area was the laundry area, a room with a series of cubby-hole boxes piled with articles of clothing. Clothing was washed in a central laundry and returned to the building. Apartments did some of their own laundry, but residents were forbidden to enter the laundry area or the staff office.

Finally, adjacent to the office in each apartment were areas for toileting and showering. The open toilets were lined up against the wall. The shower area was a large open space with a marble slab table in the center. Residents placed on the slab were sprayed and washed alternatively.

Across the hall from the living area were classrooms, offices and therapy rooms for programmed activities. Residents were wheeled there to participate in school. The hall separated where they worked and learned from where they lived. Except for the occasional trip to other parts of the building for joint activities with other groups of residents, or trips down the elevator and into an awaiting van or bus (for a medical appointment or transfer to the hospital on the grounds), the world experience of the residents was confined to two large living spaces in the apartment.

In the years between the first and the second period of observation, a new superintendent was appointed, professionals introduced programs and procedures for the implementation of the individualized educational program, and the residents of apartment M and N were dispersed to two different locations: a state mental facility – a temporary arrangement pending renovation of the building – and a new apartment located on the first floor. Seventeen of the original 53 residents lived in the new apartment. One was discharged to another institution. Another died in the hospital before I returned.

Apartment A

Apartment A had essentially the same physical layout as that of M and N (fig. 2). However, the residents were involved in programmed activities for most of the day and spent less time in the apartment or the activity area during the working hours of the professional staff. During the second phase of the research, the residents also experienced infrequent trips around the grounds of the institution and forays into the community as part of the planned and programmed school activities. Most of the residents in apartment A were not so confined to the apartment as in previous years. They experienced different environments both within and outside of the building.

The appearance of openness resulted from fewer residents in the activity area – 29 instead of 53. Fewer mats were strategically placed. The room had fewer room dividers to separate the activity area from the dining area. Dividers separated the area around the waterbed into an alcove with mats around the foot of the bed. Covering the waterbed was a sheet, the folds responding to the last person placed there. A teddy bear peeked out from underneath the pillows thrown at different angles. On either side of the waterbed rested a colored sandbag chair. In the center of the room were two other mats with cushioned triangular wedges facing one another from either side of the aisle. By the windows were rows of mats separated from each other.

Hair brushes were left on the window sill with combs stuck through them; cans of infant formula were sitting on the window sill as well as a few bowls of cereal with a half-licked spoon from the morning's breakfast. Rather than examples of unfinished work, they were evidence of "things happening." On the far side of the room in the same position and corner was a toy box piled with play things – familiar toys with which residents in the previous apartments M and N played, such as the Fisher-Price lawn mower and the rubber duck. Within the entanglements I could make out incongruous relics: a plastic garage, the arm of a crane, the side of a wooden truck, and a model Cadillac. I was astonished at the plastic guns.

A television was now located by the waterbed, with sound but no picture. It was on during the morning hours for one resident who wanted to listen. A second television console appeared but the original remained. Stereo speakers hung on the walls, the volume and the station on the radio determined by the attendants on duty. The local pop-rock station was popular with the younger attendants, but the volume was the constant concern of the apartment supervisor.

A new set of green cabinets arrived. One by one the wheelchairs and the wheelchair beds were renovated; old cracked cushions were replaced with bright shiny blue vinyl cushions. One new sign appeared: the label for "Clean" and "Dirty" over the laundry bin. It joined the other messages such as, "Mobiles are Here for the Kids!!" "When positioning the children, please try to put them within reach of a mobile and encourage him or her to play with it," "No Smoking," and "Please do not walk on

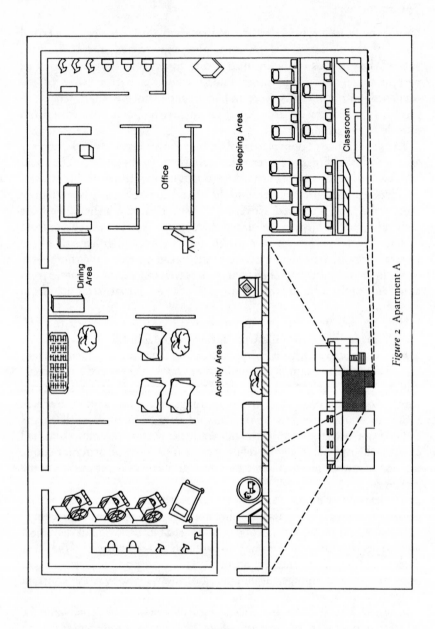

Figure 2 Apartment A

the mats." A sign on the wall identified the feeding area, the long table piled with sectioned trays, plastic bowls and cups, and specially adapted utensils. Two steel aluminum chairs were pushed in against the table and there was an office chair against the wall.

By spring 1980, residents ate in three separate locations: in the dining area in the apartment for the majority, in the classroom for individualized attention, or in the cafeteria down the hall from the apartment. The cafeteria, once used for the entire building, was for residents who could pass through a line with a tray to obtain their meal. Some residents of apartment A began eating in the cafeteria after months of improving their eating skills in the apartment. Residents from apartment A brought into the cafeteria were fed their meals while seated in their chairs around the tables of the cafeteria. The apartment remained essentially unchanged throughout the concluding months of the study except for the proliferation of notices, lists of residents involved in different groups, and schedule of trips.

On the bulletin board, in addition to the schedule of staff and their responsibilities for the day, were notices of services to be provided and the activities to be conducted throughout the week or month. Alongside the notices were occasional samples of residents' work; a card from a parent to the attendants or the teachers; notices of community trips with a list of the residents to attend. Only at the beginning of the day or in preparation for bed were the residents allowed into the sleeping area. The sleeping area was again similar to that of the other apartments but with more space for the beds and a few more photographs.

The solarium behind the sleeping area was used as a classroom during the morning and afternoon. As a classroom, the small elongated area had separate work places for different residents. Throughout the day they received a variety of medical, psychological, and therapeutic spotchecks, diagnostic interventions, and short term observations by staff. Those who participated in educational programs went to school from the activity area across the hall for approximately one-and-one-half hours each morning and afternoon. All residents participated in programmed activities if they were under 22 years of age. Residents over 22 received basic care. The apartment was less active but still a place where the residents were together when not participating in structured activities.

The timetable for the impending renovation of the building and the facilities was to follow on the heels of the reorganization of residents' classification according to functional levels (July 1977). By March 1979, the beginning of this study, the reorganization had not taken place. Building renovation scheduled for January or February of 1978 did not occur until after the residents moved from the building. The old building was not demolished until December 1981. Between my initial visit and departure from the setting (1978–79), the residents moved from apartment M and N to apartment A. Not all the residents made the same move. Some transferred to another state hospital for the mentally ill, a long-term care facility in the vicinity of the institution where the residents occupied a section of the floor in a closed and locked building of a mental hospital.

The following description found in the Title XIX records depicts the environment, personnel, and program deemed appropriate for the residents.

A small group living situation is recommended with seven to eleven other people of similar abilities. A home-like environment including sleeping, bathing, living, dining and individual and group program and activity areas each with appropriate furniture and equipment, i.e., indoor/outdoor carpeting, drapes, bedspreads, individualized chest with drawers, dining table, table cloths, couch, reclining chairs, rocking chairs, hanging lamps and indirect lighting, hanging plants, stereo and records, and educational materials.

Therapeutic use of decorations should be geared to the developmental level of the individuals with consideration of chronological age and should provide for tactile as well as visual stimulation (set at different levels on walls). Unit should be air conditioned. Also needed is a station wagon and van for transportation and an outside area for relaxation with furniture such as lawn furniture, barbecue, picnic tables.

Residential environment is required in which all staff coming into contact with the resident respond to his behavior in a structured and predetermined way. There is a predetermined system of consequences for behavior employing conditioned or primary reinforcers. Data in the form of frequency counts, response duration, and other measures is taken as a matter of course during daily activities. Training in skills and behaviors mentioned in objectives is provided by direct care and other staff using controlled stimulus presentation as delineated in written teaching programs and the ongoing system of reinforcement. Planned activities of an instructional therapeutic or recreational nature are happening in the residence during a large majority of those hours in which residents are awake and not in programs outside of the residence.

Staffing would include an Apartment Director (a professional, serving as Program Coordinator) who reports directly to a Program Director. The Apartment Director would supervise direct care staff over three shifts in programmatic and personal care programs as well as administratively supervise and schedule daily input of professional staff. All staff, other than consultants, will be assigned full time working a minimum of 32 hours per week directly with residents and training staff out of this program setting, (special arrangements being made to assure that part of daily program is carried out, outside of residential setting) 8 hours a week would be set for planning, meetings, professional inservice, etc. Professional staff ratio as specific as in evaluation. Direct care staff ratio of 1:3 during waking hours at all times, 1:8 during sleeping hours. (Title XIX Evaluation, 1975)

The accent was on the need for professional services to monitor the residents' condition, develop programs, design accommodations within the environment, make adaptations to wheelchairs and stretcher beds, procure special equipment, and structure resident interaction with the use of behavior modification. The answer to the overcrowding and the overstimulation in the apartments was new home-like environments. Increasingly, the present building was cited for deficiencies in the recent federal and state inspections. For example, adaptive toilets were needed but there would be no immediate replacement or adaptation until the renovation. Staff were told the problems would be solved by "remodelling."

Gradually over the three years the residents were moved from the apartment to the individualized classrooms for programs. A quiet environment, free from distractions from learning, was a reality by 1980.

The population

You got to know them [residents] to identify them. In an institution they have to have an identity of their own. (Attendant, 1980)

The institution was founded as a school to serve the needs of the handicapped in the greater metropolitan area of a large urban center. The archive records provide a general description of the residents. These demographic data reveal the diversity in the population of residents in terms not only of their handicaps but also of their backgrounds. They are not a group of individuals from one neighborhood, or geographical area, or local school. They have come to live together in this apartment for the care the institution provides.

The clinical description is based on a series of examinations and evaluations. The first step, "impressions at admission," includes formal and informal clinical reports from other agencies and parental records. Completing this review, the examining physician identifies clinical characteristics in a "provisional diagnosis." These characteristics and impressions in part determine temporary placement in the institution. Medical statements describe the level and the prognosis for the individual. An "established diagnosis" of functional level follows a complete series of evaluations and assessments by staff professionals during the first months and years in the institution. Some examiners received different impressions and experienced problems in gaining a full evaluation. The notations by the attendants and the professionals came to constitute what was known of the resident. While personal impressions of the resident might contrast, the clinical impressions of a resident's condition were consistent, although comments became more systematic and analytic after the Title XIX evaluations of the mid 1970s. In recent evaluations of residents, a list of "master problems" is based on case studies and evaluations. These lists describe, in short simple statements, what the resident can and cannot do

29

across all areas of functioning. This new shorthand replaces clinical labels and objectives.

The archive records reveal no specific clinical category by which to define the population. A complicated array of physical handicaps constrained most areas of an individual's functioning. The profound levels of mental retardation resulted in impairment to the sensory modalities, modifying the processing of information and affecting cognition. Many individuals were subject to random and debilitating disturbances of the central nervous system. In this setting, the medical and psychological consensus was encapsulated in the clinical label of "severely and profoundly mentally retarded and multiply handicapped." The label referred to the stable and uncompromising nature of multiple handicaps that necessitated total care and supervision throughout a lifetime. The residents had not developed the skills of self-maintenance: they were unable to feed, dress, bathe, or in some cases, move themselves.

Background information

Among the 64 residents were equal numbers of males and females. The majority were voluntary admissions from parents, family members and legally appointed guardians. One came from a foster home and one through the courts. Two were born outside the United States. Twenty of the parents had admitted a family member after a prolonged series of hospital visits or short-term trips to the institution. Sixteen came directly from the hospital, three from other institutions and five from the public schools.

The age of admission was relatively young; 47 were under 15 years when admitted with one exception, aged 25 years. The average age throughout the three years of the study was 21 years in January 1978, and 24 years in June 1980. At the completion of the study in June 1980, the youngest was nine years of age and the oldest 60. Most were in their mid-twenties.

Reasons for the admissions during the late 1950s and the early 1960s included a view of the child as too big to carry or to handle, inability to follow the programs that were offered, and exhaustion. Parents sought quantifiable evidence of the degree and level of retardation before admission. Some were prepared for the obvious handicaps – they had accepted the blindness, for instance – but were not prepared for the inability to walk. Others felt frustration with the fact that they themselves were not able to provide therapy at an early age, or with contradictory medical opinions. Forty of the residents came from the counties around the institutional and the metropolitan area. Once admitted to the institution, most of the residents were placed in apartment M or N immediately.

The population

Only three began their institutionalization in other buildings and locations on the grounds. Placement in the building and in the apartment was definitive. Once placed in the apartment the resident was not going to move elsewhere.

By June 1980, the average length of stay in the institution was 19 years, the shortest stay to date five years, and the longest, 46 years. Over the three years, two were discharged to another institution and one moved to a community residence to participate in a secondary vocational public school program. Two deaths occurred, one during the observation period of an undiagnosed and untreatable infection, and the second after the period of formal observation, from continuous respiratory problems.

Clinical classification

Medical and psychological descriptions of the residents are clinical designations which portray the stability and the uncompromising nature of the handicaps. The most recent information is from the clinical abstracts and the profile of the client.

The general classification of "mentally deficient" appears to be the first diagnosis on the records of those admitted the earliest to the institution. Mental deficiency was supplanted later by more sophisticated and precise clinical syndrome categories and by psychological and behavioral terms: for example, "mental retardation – severe or profound."

At admission, 21 residents were considered profoundly mentally retarded and 11 severely mentally retarded. For 16 of the residents, the category shifted from severe to profound mental retardation in the years following admission. Once the label "profound mental retardation" was attached in more recent years, no change in classification occurred. Only five of the residents reversed the downward spiral from severe to profound, suggesting that they possessed greater ability than was first assumed. The residents as a group, however, were considered to be at the lower end of the spectrum of mental retardation.

Fifteen different medical categories found in the records describe the residents. No individuals belong to more than nine out of the 15 categories. The majority (33) share complications of spasticity; brain damage; micro-, hydro-, or macrocephaly; musculoskeletal problems; and epilepsy (33). Other complications were with the sensory modalities (27), cerebral palsy (6), heart (3), spine (23), and neurological insults (7). While degree and complexity of handicap varied, the overriding nature of the organic origin and nature of these categories was systematically documented in the records.

The cause of mental retardation is not easy to pinpoint. The compound nature of the cerebral and the central nervous system disturbance makes a precise designation difficult. Congenital problems were the identified cause of mental retardation for 28 of the residents. For 17 residents the cause was questionable or unknown. The surprising fact is that relatively few exemplify a specific cause, that is, only nine had an identified metabolic or genetic disorder. General causes cited were anoxia (10); trauma before, during, or after the birth process (9); and prematurity (8). Injury after the birth process was due, in one case, to accident, and in the other, to battered child syndrome.

Intelligence tests administered to residents between 1953 and 1977 were the Gesell, Leiter, and Peabody tests, and the Wechsler Intelligence Scale for Children. Three individuals were labeled "untestable" after extensive evaluations between 1975 and 1977. Most of the residents participated in testing with multiple trials if the examiner was unable to obtain a result. Those who obtained scores include 48 profoundly mentally retarded (IQ of 20 or less); seven severely mentally retarded (IQ of 20–35); one each in categories of mild (IQ 52–67) and borderline (IQ between 68–83). Seven had no psychological numerical determination.

Labeling and testing of intelligence were supplanted by a categorical behavioral distinction. For individuals admitted between 1952 and 1957, the primary descriptive terms used were "institutional," "idiot," "improbable," and "incontinent." "Institutional" and "idiot" are not terms in use today.

The current behavioral terms applied to the population include "averbal," "non-ambulatory," "self abusive," "social problem," "toilet care," and "total care." Fifteen residents bore one label, averbal. Eighteen required total care. Fifteen exhibited social problems and two were self-abusive, and four required specific behavioral management in the environment. Five walked independently; 29 were confined to a wheelchair and 25 to a bed stretcher. Three were learning to walk with assistance. During the period of the study, the categories did not change.

Originally, the residents in the building were to have received specialized training for sensory handicaps, in addition to a program for mental retardation. Twenty-seven of the residents had sensory handicaps, requiring sensory stimulation. Twenty-nine required constant medical treatment on the ward and one required geriatric accommodations.

In terms of daily living and the ability to care for their personal and bodily needs, the census indicates that 58 had no toilet ability, and only three had accomplished toilet training; 38 needed to be fed while 20 required assistance; 52 were unable to dress themselves and 10 required partial assistance. Forty-eight did not communicate through any recognized medium, seven relied on gestures and three on signs, and two had a single word or phrase. These categories did not change in the reports during the three years of the study.

Twenty-two of the residents received no medication in 1981, the comparison of the last reported dosage show the remainder receiving an average of 3.5 pills per day. For 22 of the residents this represents a decrease in medication by an average of three pills per day between 1978 and 1981. For another 22 there was an average increase of three pills per day. Twenty-four different medications fell into four categories: aid to elimination (44), anti-convulsants (36), vitamin-supplements (15), and anti-psychotic drugs (14). Seventeen of the residents received a general medication for a temporary condition. There was a decrease in the use of anti-psychotic drugs, a continuous use of anti-convulsants, particularly for the management of epilepsy, and an increase in the use of medication to promote elimination.

The residents: an introduction

On each trip to the institution over the month of discussions with the assistant superintendent which preceded my research at the institution, I watched the residents walk along the side of the road on the drive to the administration building. As I watched, each resident would stop, turn and face the car, and wave. Some clutched a pocketbook in one hand, others a pipe. One would hum the melody of a tune; another, muttering a string of obscenities directed at a boss in the workshop, increased volume as someone approached. Others were lost in conversation with themselves, or walked silently hand-in-hand with another resident. Sometimes the driver of the car stopped to say hello. In general the questions asked were "What's your name?" "Where do you work?" "What building are you in?" "Do you have a smoke?" The conversation always ended with a cheerful wave as both driver and the resident acknowledged that they had to go to work. On the bridge over a little stream along the back driveway to the school, three men with lunch pails sat smoking their corncob pipes.[2]

A woman dressed in a large red coat which brushed against the top of her boots walked mumbling to herself. Another man with a radio to his ear watched her. The path from the lunchroom swerved down to the bottom of a small incline, where water from the melting snow collected to form a large puddle over the path. She stopped and started to yell and curse the puddle, "Why is this f——— stream here for?" "Why is this stream here?" "What is this f——— puddle?" She stopped and looked around and yelled all the louder repeating the same questions. There was silence. Then without trying to walk around it, yelling curses but no longer asking questions, she stepped into the puddle.

Two adults passed, commenting on her situation and said directly to her, "Heh, you can't have it easy every day of your life." They walked around the band of ice that separated the snow and the water. They passed on with the comment, neither staying to watch her nor clarifying the statement. She waded into the puddle. She stopped at the very deepest and yelled at the top of her lungs, "This damn puddle!"

She stood in the center of the puddle cursing the Almighty for putting this puddle in her path. As I walked into the administration building, I glanced over my shoulder as she emerged from the other side continuing on her way, dragging her oversize boots along the pavement.

There were other instances of a woman or a man dressed in white, pulling along a resident as he sucked his thumb and screamed, trying to walk in the direction opposite to that of the hand that was trying to guide him. Or the resident who was just getting off her shift at the workshop laughing at the resident who was going to replace her and commanding, "Get to work!" Often the older resident took charge of the others, as if in imitation of what she herself had experienced, rounding a few stragglers into line and saying, "Come on now, time to go home. Keep moving." The pace was always tediously slow, and each part of the sequence of movement a snapshot in a string of pictures.

I entered the building for the first time during this transition from a period when residents were isolated in buildings according to syndrome and categorical level to the new groupings based on skill and ability. As I waited outside the office of the unit director, glancing at a bulletin board display of a winter scene, I watched a large woman in a disheveled wig limp down the hall shifting her weight while pushing the wheelchair stretcher. From the stretcher peered a tiny white face over a gigantic oversized bib tied to her neck, surrounded by pillows, her legs entwined in the sheets that covered the stretcher and her torso. The tips of her fingers flickered up and down rapidly through the tunnel that her arm made in the sheet. The woman fell heavily into a chair, swinging the stretcher around in front of her. She looked down at the white face, wiped the drool from her chin and mouth, and looked up and over to me. We stared alternately at one another and at the pale little face in the sea of white sheets.

Another "grandmother" volunteer with another resident appeared from down the hall.

"How is Pamela today?"
"Good," was the reply.
"How is yours?"
"Excited and moving about," came the reply.

And they gradually drifted into conversations about the transportation problems of going back and forth to work.

I met the building psychologist, who was to oversee the study and coordinate relationships with other members of the staff. He was to be the only person to remain attentive to the study throughout the years of research.

The residents: an introduction

"I am really glad you're interested in studying our clients. Few staff members believe that these individuals do anything. We are at the bottom of the barrel in terms of the other residents in the institutions. Everyone thinks that they [the residents] are just so bad off that they don't really deserve anything. They do more than people know. You get to like and enjoy them after you're here for a while."

We began a tour of the building and my first meeting with the residents. We passed through the doors to meet the familiar odor of urine or disinfectant. The first ward with its cardboard sign, apartment A, was in physical terms just like the last.

In apartment A, I watched the attendants lift a limp body into a sandbag chair. He was heavy and just made it over the ridge of the chair into the hole pounded into its center. The older attendant sighed, "Phew, we got him into the chair." As we passed on, the psychologist stopped and looked down at Melissa sitting in her wheelchair. He leaned on the arm of the wheelchair. He leaned on the arm of the wheelchair and looked at the distance from Melissa's foot to the footrest. "We've got to get this wheelchair adjusted to her size again." He stared at the woman's face. Melissa extended her hand slowly and deliberately upward. The psychologist shook her hand saying, "What's the matter?" We moved on.

Apartment C came up quickly. The psychologist said, "These residents are from another building. They have a really bad reputation from over there. These are toilet-trained and they are at the sensory stimulation and awareness level."

Five clients were in the activity area with three people standing around looking at one individual in a sandbag chair. No one stopped their conversation or their observation of a resident, but they glanced at us. Another attendant moved May over onto another mat and placed a mobile over her head and dropped it down to a level for May to hit. She smiled as this was being done. She hit it again and laughed.

"This is behavior management/basic skills. They need behavior management because they throw furniture, break windows and strip, and all need toilet-training," the psychologist said as we all entered apartment D. One man in a tee shirt and long khaki trousers surrounding his feet immediately came up to me and shook hands. "How are you, buddy?" He did not look at me or pause, but kept walking over to another resident and sat by him. The psychologist directed my attention to a group of men walking in circles and said, "These are blind." I was surprised from their movement. Others rolled on the beds and babbled. Staff attendants watched from their chairs, sitting some men down, standing others up.

Apartment E was different. A number of individuals were in chairs, lying on the floor and on mats. Besides the large man sitting on the back of the chair twirling a cowboy hat, there were four older women who went to each individual, cooing and tickling and laughing in their faces. "How are you today?" A bright smile rose over the features of one boy's face as he stiffened and then jerked his entire body in response to the greeting. The woman then went on to the next individual with her same set of routines and greetings. The psychologist was standing at the side of the crib asking,

"How are you today?"

He turned to me.

"This is Gertie. Macrocephalic ... Everyone is sympathetic to her. She is alert. Yes, she knows everything. She understands. But she has gone downhill. The crib in the rear was made special for her so she could see through the glass."

I walked back to see the crib in the solarium. In the warmth of the sun lay a woman trying to take off the rest of her clothing. She struggled with pulling her dress over her head. I brought it to the psychologist's attention by staring. He walked back and remarked.

"Oh yes, that's Mary. It's real hard to keep clothes on her. She does that to everything we put on her. She's impossible."

We left her in the struggle. We went upstairs to a newly refurbished apartment O. It smelled heavily of ammonia. I was glad of the break in the sights, sounds, and smells as we walked upstairs. Inside apartment O, the physical setting was refreshing by comparison. A male attendant stood in the middle of a crowd of residents walking in circles, milling around him. The television was on but no one appeared to be watching. Lying on the floor in the middle was a young man with black hair who had a smile on his face as if enjoying the company of others' feet. No one paid attention to him, but no one stepped on him either. I looked down at the floor and realized he was staring at me. I looked; he continued to stare. I winked; he stared. I winked again; he stared. I winked my other eye; he stared. I winked again; he watched intently and smiled. I winked the opposite eye and he focused on my eyes. I switch-winked very fast. He laughed out loud so hard that his whole body shook. I walked away wondering, "What has just happened?" As the psychologist passed through the doors into the next room, we passed into an empty room, vacant because of repainting. "The residents in this bedroom will share jointly the activity area for apartment M. This is N." And we walked through another door into the far end of a large playroom.

The activity area, or play area, was shared jointly by residents of apartments M and N. The room was larger than any activity area we had seen so far. Residents were everywhere. We carefully made our way through gymnastic mats and bodies on the floor. I would catch sight of a head and a leg and a hand from under the sheets, diapers and bibs and pillows surrounding each client. Some clients slumped into depressions in sandbag chairs. The mounds of sand in the chair fit their contours, supporting a variety of shapes and angles.

For all the stillness, there seemed to be a tremendous commotion in the activity area. I smiled as I caught sight of Benjamin sitting in a rocking chair at the other end of a row of mats from which I had just come. With one leg propped up to rest its foot on the opposite knee, and the other leg lifting up and down on the floor to rock the chair, he leaned back in the rocker and smiled and gurgled and grunted in a stream of sunlight. He seemed to be watching the whole area, overseeing everyone on the floor. (Benjamin is blind. I retained my first impression, that he could see, for two more visits.) Another client prone on a stretcher stared at the ceiling, turning his head back and forth occasionally. An attendant walking by on her way to change another resident, lifted the rolled diaper in her hand and said, "Stop that Donald!" Donald had his hands in his diaper. The psychologist turned to me and said, "This is where you might want to be." The tour was complete in my own mind. It was here I wanted to stay.

The psychologist tried to find the apartment supervisor. In the office of the apartment supervisor, I explained that I would like to observe the social interaction in the activity area.

She said, "Oh, that's interesting. There are chairs who run over the others. Here we have to keep the wheelchairs separated from the crawlers."

I said quickly, "Yes that's it! That's what I want to study." To me this meant, not only that the residents would do something but also that staff would intervene in their activity.

The programs

Programs were mandated by federal and state law. Assessment, examination, and determination of unique needs and abilities captured a profile of the individual from which the educational program developed. The programs implemented over the three years of this study evolved during the *process* of meeting resident needs. The process involved two sets of individuals: professional and direct care staff. The attendants provided basic care on a daily basis. They fed, showered, changed, diapered, made beds, did laundry, administered snacks and liquid supplements, and supervised residents during the rest period. The professional staff assessed, examined, determined individual needs, and conducted lessons and therapy.

The logistics of coordinating the provision of services for a number of residents with increasing case loads became a significant issue for all staff. The professionals made weighty decisions for care of the residents, knowing there was little opportunity to provide all that was needed. Description of programs for the residents laid out the ideal: the best possible service. The ideal competed with the reality of staff limitations, scheduling problems, and actual delivery of service to each of the 64 residents. The resulting frustration, however, never resulted in more than a request for more staff to provide the necessary services.

Supervision and coordination of the programs in the building rested with the psychologist. After the annual review, the psychologist observed the actual progress of the residents in these programs. The psychologist oversaw and coordinated the implementation of programs by the professionals.

In 1980, an educational coordinator was appointed to administer the delivery of teachers' services. Supervision of other professionals rested with the department within the institution. Significantly, the department of physical therapy supervised the planning, coordination, and implementation of the physical therapy program and the therapists. Thus, while the professionals conducted the residents' programs in the apartment, they were supervised from outside the building. The professionals interpreted practice and programs by reference to their peers. Practice reflected the experience, the judgment, and the resources of the individual professional.

The opportunity to offer coordinated systematic programs to the severely and profoundly mentally retarded and the multiply handicapped was both a goal and a dream for the staff. Educational and therapeutic programs had not previously been available to this population. Programs to meet the resident needs were designed by professional staff to stimulate the sense modalities, to provide medical care and supervision, and to manage behavior. Young professionals found themselves face-to-face with the reality of being in charge of programs for the residents. Staff who had worked with the severely and profoundly mentally retarded and multiply handicapped, or within this particular building, found themselves to be valuable resources because of their familiarity with the residents. The 1978–79 school year saw professionals refer to themselves as specialists. The teacher of previous years was now the educational specialist; the teacher who conducted a behavior modification program in a classroom became the behavior management specialist.

Professionals with experience moved away from providing direct care and service within the educational programs to consultation in the specialist role. Teachers with one or two aides conducted selected exercises with the residents, at the same time managing the direction and supervision of aides. This general movement removed a number of professionals from direct delivery of services. For example, the behavior management specialist became a roving consultant, responsible for behavior programs with residents and on call for troubles in other programs. Teaching was complicated by supervision of aides, consultation, management of program delivery, and maintenance of records – for example, the problem of communicating performance criteria to aides conducting the activity. Skill sheets were often filled out by the aide conducting the lesson, but the final reports and quarterly reports were written and signed by the teacher or educational program coordinator. The records are a mix of specific lessons conducted by staff on a one-to-one basis and more general statements made after a group lesson in the activity area. The records show an increase in professionals in the setting and a wide variety of programs provided by specialists, with numerous opinions of resident performance and standardization of criteria relating to behavioral objectives.

The professionals determined individual needs first by the evaluation and assessment of the individual across all dimensions of intellectual, social, physical, and developmental domains. On this basis a professional with expertise in a particular domain identified areas of need in activities of daily living or socialization. A program in that need area was designed – for example, to teach the individual how to dress or to teach interaction with peers. Within the context of the program, the professional delineated associated skills, defined in terms of specific behaviors within the lesson – for example, to pull on a shirt, or to reach toward and touch a peer.

In a program, staff conducted an activity to achieve a predetermined objective for a skill. Skills were ordered in a linear progression through a normal developmental sequence. Progress from programs within the institution to mainstream life necessitated movement through functional levels – for example, vertical movement through the levels of sensory stimulation and basic skills to vocational; or, lateral movement across levels of medical, geriatric, communication, and behavior management when the individual's needs in these areas demanded attention or over-rode skill development on other levels. Within functional designations, a skill or skill level was organized progressively toward more "appropriate" behavior. Skill mastery meant not only progression to another skill level, but also movement to another apartment. Skills and associated behaviors became competences which determined the individual's residence within the institution.

Individuals were grouped according to their areas of need or functional level. For example, the residents of this building and apartment were at "sensory stimulation," the first functional level. For residents identified at this functional level, the professional staff first determined what the residents could do through a series of examinations and assessments conducted in the apartment by watching their bathing, dressing, and feeding routines. Assessments and evaluation continued with initiation of educational activities and therapy sessions. Then staff set priorities for programs, for example to develop self-awareness and awareness of their environment.

The residents lived with other residents in need of sensory experiences to enhance development. Sensory experiences were the first developmental level in the institutional organization. It was the level from which no resident could be excluded for non-performance. Progress in the sensory areas meant response to activities and lessons leading to the introduction of other skills in a developmental approach to assessment and organization (De Grandpre, 1973). Participation in the sensory motor experiences – fine and gross motor, bathing, feeding, and community experience – was the focus, with an emphasis on the development of skills necessary for survival. Presumably, these are prerequisite skills required to function with others. In peer interaction and socialization programs pairs of residents learned to touch each other, roll a ball, or pass an object to each other. Staff selected the pairs of residents for the activity and the ease

39

Table 2. *Schedule of resident programs*

Time	Apartment location	Program
6:30–7:30	Sleeping area	Wake-up, dressing
7:30–8:30	Activity area: dining section	Breakfast
8:30–9:30	Activity area	Showering Activities of daily living Medications
9:30–10:00	Activity area	Transition to school Transportation to clinics
10:00–11:30	Activity area	Positioning program
	Classrooms and therapy room	School programs
11:30–12:00	Activity area	Transition to activity area
12:00–1:00	Activity area: dining section	Lunch
1:00–1:45	Activity area	Rest period
1:45–2:15	Activity area	Change of diapers Medications Transition to school
2:15–3:00	Activity area	Positioning program
	Classroom and therapy room	School programs
3:00–3:30	Activity area	Transition to activity area
3:30–4:30	Activity area	Positioning in activity area
4:30–5:00	Activity area	Preparation for mealtime
5:00–6:15	Activity area: dining section	Dinner
6:15–7:00	Activity area	Preparation for bed Activities of daily living Medications Television
7:00–8:00	Sleeping area	Bed

with which it was accomplished determined staff involvement. A developmental approach to assessment and programming for the residents was a short-term goal on the road to normalization and deinstitutionalization.

The physical structure of the building provided the boundary between the institution and the world outside it. For the residents, their world view and experience come from within those walls. Before 1975, the program for the residents described in reports consisted of feeding, showering, activities of daily living, and positioning: activities to keep the residents clean, dry, healthy, and safe throughout the three years of this study (see table 2). The schedule in the records was fixed, but in reality it was fluid and variable, depending on staff changes in shifts, lunch and coffee breaks, and staff meetings. The residents were handled interchangeably by attendants, professionals, and their aides. Aides were often reassigned from one individual to another. Attendants rotated the showering, changing, and bedmaking almost daily. All shared equally in the care both of residents who were enjoyable to work with and of those who presented problems. Moving or lifting a resident, especially one of the heavier ones, was not greeted with enthusiasm by anyone on the staff, but all worked within the schedule and towards fulfilling its demands.

After the initiation of resident evaluations, a subtle shift in the definition of a program occurred. Positioning was a case in point. Positioning describes a period of the day – usually two hours in the morning, after shower and before lunch, or after rest period for two hours in the afternoon after lunch – when the residents were laid out on the mats, settled in sandbag chairs, or propped up in triangular wedges. Attendants supervised them from chairs about the room. Residents could watch the attendants and the other staff pass by, wave, say hello, tickle them or throw a toy to them, as they moved about the apartment doing their chores, folding the laundry or making the beds. They could watch the nurse, in a white clinic jacket with a stethoscope around her neck, pushing a cart with vials of medication. They could watch the psychologist, in sport shirt and knit tie, carrying a clipboard and stopwatch, take a seat on the mat to time behavior.

In 1978, the positioning program involved rotating the residents to change their positions. The activity was similar; a therapeutic rationale was provided.

Anita has quite a bit of mobility and can move herself around when allowed to do so. She sits nicely in a beanbag chair with her head back and this allows her to look around. She should always be sitting upright as possible to prevent further scoliosis.

Anita reaches and grasps with her left hand so toys or any kind of stimuli should be placed on her left side. Noise makers, music, eye contact, and feeling different textures are good stimulation for her. (Positioning program, 1978)

The description became a prescription for positioning in a programmatic sense. Similar programming extended to feeding, bathing, dressing, music, recreation, activities of daily living, washing, range-of-motion, and toilet.

Before 1977, six residents had participated in 20 different programs. By 1977 the number of programs had grown to 30, including such additions as peer interaction, foster-grandparents, orthopedic ambulation, and tutoring. The foster-grandparent program assigned an elderly caretaker to an individual for a portion of the day. 'Orthopedic' meant that an orthopedic specialist evaluated the residents' orthopedic needs and developed an ambulation program. The year 1978 saw 47 different program areas mushroom for the 64 residents. The number of programs gradually decreased due to changes in the setting, including the transfer of residents outside of the building.

After 1977, more residents participated in each program. In 1978, 56 residents were involved in a feeding program, 47 in sensory stimulation, 37 in music, 27 in educational classes, and 23 in recreation. The quarantine imposed on the building curtailed some services during 1979. In 1980 the number of program areas was 29, with a substantial reduction in the number of participating residents. Professional involvment in evaluation and provision of programs remained strongest during 1978–80.

In 1978, the programs became more than activities of daily living: they became any area of professional involvement or intervention in the lives of the residents, from feeding and nutrition to the differentiation of gross and fine motor skills, participation in educational classroom activities, socialization, recreation, and peer interaction.

On a daily basis, a teacher or aide conducted activities with a resident from a specific lesson plan. Given a particular need area (for example, the need for socialization), the teacher developed a lesson to teach a particular objective: "The resident will roll a ball a distance of one foot to another resident four out of five times." The teacher placed the residents side-by-side a foot apart, rolled the ball to them, and said, "Roll the ball, Thomas, roll the ball Danial." The teacher rolled the ball in the right direction, correcting its course if necessary; ensured that the ball was within the grasp of the other resident; and offered exclamations and praise if the residents coordinated movement to hit the ball or made any effort to pass it between them. The teacher maintained the activity for as long as the residents participated, or encouraged participation beyond what they were inclined to do. If the objective was met, the teacher annotated the record. If not, the teacher planned more practice the following day, or more likely, the next time that socialization group occurred. At the end of the week, their progress determined whether or not the activity should be continued. The teacher might change the ball, substitute another object, try participation with another resident. The program changed accordingly during the conduct of the lesson, the school day, or when teacher and aide discussed the resident.

Each week the teacher planned new activities and objectives for each individual for the following week. At the end of the month, the performance of the resident on objectives, along with the remarks of teacher or aides, were registered on a chart which was the basis for the next monthly plan.

The programs

These daily, weekly, and monthly records fed quarterly reviews in which objectives in all the areas of resident performance were reviewed and revised. Supervisors read quarterly reviews to check the objectives for the residents. These quarterly reports, the lesson plans, and the progress notes formed the basis of the annual review for each resident. The annual review gathered all the professionals involved with the one individual resident and covered all aspects of the individual's life. At the annual review, a general review of the resident's status and the delivery of services was discussed. An individualized educational program was developed. For each of the 64 residents, professionals determined programs and participation in any of 47 activity areas and the need for further evaluations, assessments, and reports. The formal measure by which progress of the residents was recorded was progress on the objective.

Other documents provided information. Formal reports and evaluations described performance during an evaluation; progress notes of the professional or the attendant in the course of the day described the condition of the resident. The schedule of activities provided information on the consistency of a particular program over time. In conjunction with the lesson plans and objectives, a clear picture emerged of what the resident actually did in program areas over the three year period.

Program areas were scheduled activities arranged by the professional staff for a specific resident after a determination of his or her individual needs at the annual review. The purpose of the activity and the lesson in a program area was to teach the specific skill, or to acquaint the individual with the skill area. In the area of communication, a lesson might include attempts to encourage the resident to respond to a greeting such as "Good morning," to point to – or otherwise indicate recognition of – an object or picture, or to learn the sign language for specific expressions. The name for a program could be ambiguous: sometimes it indicated what the resident did, and sometimes it indicated what was done to them. For example, the name of the mealtime activity was "feeding," not "eating." Why not "mealtime," or "mealtime – breakfast"?

Leisure, recreation and peer interaction suggested a similar activity in a program area. Leisure was a quiet time when the residents were left on their own. Recreation included activities found under the headings of leisure time, peer interaction and socialization, and play, for example, rolling a ball between peers. In programs the activity was also prescribed. In a relaxation program the professionals sought to "relax the client" through a series of rubbings, holdings, and pattings. The professional judged the degree of relaxation. Skills to be developed in an activity were also predetermined for program areas. The emphasis was on the acquisition of skills and the activities were a means to that end.

Socialization as a program area was incorporated into the individual schedule of teachers in the fall of 1977 and as a primary program area during 1979–80. Socialization indicated participation and intervention in social ways with other severely and profoundly mentally retarded and multiply handicapped individuals. The socialization group taught socialization skills that were developmentally and culturally appropriate even though expectations were adjusted. (Residents' behavior in the apartment on their own could be compared with their behavior in lessons designed to teach them social behavior.) In the fall of 1979 a joint socialization group formed after peer interaction was curtailed or minimized during the quarantine (1978–79).

Community involvement of the residents increased throughout 1980, especially in the area of recreation. Staff were eager to involve the residents in experiences in the immediate metropolitan area of the institution. Eating in restaurants, shopping trips, visits to exhibits, museums, local fairs and carnivals, as well as public appearances at the symphony concert, were scheduled as part of their educational experience.

The case study is developed as a history of the individual's participation within programs offered and is a picture of the skills and abilities observed by staff. Skill categories and levels of achievement for residents are standardized and performance criteria are set. Behavioral objectives become the means for reporting resident achievement on skills across all program areas. All the information about the resident in programs is assembled into this case study. Comments considered derogatory or opinionated are dropped.

Determination of a program begins with an examination which consists of a professional watching performance on a designated activity. The music therapist puts a tamborine into the hands of the resident and sings and plays a tune, waiting for a response. The teacher introduces educational tasks such as sorting beads, picture cards, or blocks. The behavior specialist asks the resident to do something, and tests a "reinforcer" such as M&M candy or cookies or popcorn. The adaptive equipment wheelchair specialist asks the resident to reach down to the wheel of the chair, to move feet onto foot pedals to determine if the seat, wheel, or pedals need adjustment. The physical therapist expects the resident to roll over or to move in a particular direction upon command. Reports identify these situations and include a short description of what the examiner asks the resident to do, and what the examiner finds. Statements vary in form and content. Medical eye-and-ear reports give levels of vision and hearing. Physical therapy reports focus on clinical description and prognosis for the function of muscles. The educator identifies skills related to eye–hand coordination, cognitive skills, and visual–motor integration. The behavior specialist describes ability to attend, to follow directions, and to respond to reinforcement. Individual reports conclude with recommendations.

The reporting format includes: (1) a statement of the examination conducted, (2) the tasks and test, and items administered, (3) assessment of performance on the tasks, (4) recommendations within the area of functioning, and (5) prognosis. Assessments can overlap on general skills, such as the ability to attend, or they may be specific to the particular discipline. The skills are isolated as separate entities, removed from the context of performance. Interpretation and integration into manageable programs are left to teachers and practitioners.

Sometimes it is difficult to see the relationship between one skill and another; the reports do not make explicit the relationship between task and lesson, or between lesson and skill development. The question remains whether these relations and links are clear even in "normal" individuals, let alone in the severely or profoundly mentally retarded and the multiply handicapped with their complicated and interrelated handicaps. These case studies constitute the data from which program priorities are determined for the year.

The annual review is the occasion when priorities for a resident – based on the case study – are set. All reports and progress on objectives are considered at this time. Goals include provision of service, development of skills, including "leisure time" skills, maintenance of involvement, and prevention of further degeneration. One resident, Rex, had a total of 29 need areas for which goals were set and programs assigned. Need areas are associated with specific disciplines and professional orientation. For instance, the recreation specialist helps Rex develop leisure time activities in the need area of companionship; social services seeks a tutor to act as a companion. The annual review identifies the optimal program for the individual. For Rex's 29 need areas, a professional or an agency is designated to meet the need.

An endless search for more people to help across all areas is reflected in the 64 individual reports. Individual assistance depends on the availability of the professional to provide the service and on the workability of a schedule. Companionship is treated, not simply in terms of companions (other residents), but in terms of a normal adult providing stimulating interaction with the resident. The more needs that are identified, the more focused and fragmented the interpretation of examinations and the resulting programs. Needs are identified on an individual basis, independent of the ability to provide the service; then they are ranked in order of priority for incorporation into the program. The records are an historical document of what professionals define as resident needs and they ensure professional accountability.

The years 1979–80 saw increased emphasis on consultation – professional opinion on status and the progress of the resident and determination of appropriate placement and programs for the resident inside and outside of the institution.

The standardization of programs formalized the roles of and relationships between the attendants and the professional staff, especially the teachers. Attendants provided the basic care, professionals taught, and specialists acted as consultants.

Martin appears to be in good spirits, toys are available for him to play with and continually played with him during the visit. I am available for consultation for anything that might come up regarding Martin. Please continue the concerned efforts which all staff are making to keep Martin active. If he becomes inactive, he will pick up self stimulating behaviors. Thank you. (Psychologist, 1979)

Due to inconsistent staff coverage, supervision, and lack of apartment organization, I am temporarily discontinuing noting any further progress or lack of it until some consistency is directed towards the apartment and its clients. Kenneth did not meet his annual objective of ADL [activities of daily living] skills. If anyone is interested in continuing a program with much needed consistency, I will be available for consultation on Kenneth. ADL – Bathing and Dressing Procedures are found in the "Pattern of Care" section of his record. (Psychologist, 1979)

Beginning in September 1979 with the implementation of programs for the residents, the professional staff supervised less and less of the residents' day-to-day life in the apartment because of their increasing involvement in programs. The residents' involvement in programmed activities for most of the morning and afternoon precluded contact with the basic care staff except during rest period. The attendants became less and less involved in seeing and learning about what the professionals were doing because of the separation of their duties. This is a significant shift from the first phase of the research, during which a majority of the residents remained in the apartment throughout the day, and during which some of the lessons and activities were actually conducted in the activity area itself, where the attendants could watch and participate in the activity.

This shift in participation, along with the schedule of breaks, mealtimes, and shift changes, endangered an already fragile relationship. The attendants learned about what the residents did from the professionals. In 1979, only the rest period remained as a time when the attendants and the residents were together during the daytime shifts. Thus supervision by attendants took the form of spot checks when a problem arose, or when a resident's screaming became irksome.

During rest period, all the residents were taken from their wheelchairs and stretcher beds (with a very few exceptions) and settled onto mats. Residents were left alone for the most part, their activities and adventures constrained only by attendants returning them to mats, separating them from one another, or removing toys. At the end of the rest period, diapers were changed and afternoon lessons begun. Teachers returned to find residents under sheets, nestled with toys, or hugging one another. Attendants or the staff made few notes about the rest period.

Although some of the attendants initiated play activities with the residents in 1978, these encounters by attendant staff noticeably declined in 1979 and 1980. In this way, attendants came to perform only the minimum requirements of the job – basic care and supervision – interacting only occasionally with favorite residents, while the professional staff interacted with the residents in a programmed and structured way. Spontaneity in the interaction with the residents dwindled not only in notations in the records by attendants, but in observations in the wards during the second phase of the research (1979–80).

A critical problem of such observation and reporting of the residents' interaction and participation with each other and with staff is the absence of context. Simply said, what the staff see and what the residents do is not fully reported. Examination and assessment do not exclude a concern with the whole individual, but the complexity of what is being observed is reduced to what is an identifiable fragment of behavior. Not reported in formal objectives and clinical case studies is tacit information – for example spontaneous moments of play, the assignment of a nickname, the observation of a unique behavior by a resident. Engagement with the residents requires a spontaneous interaction attentive to the subtleties of their behavior. The clinical case study, on the other hand, demands a positivistic, objective report on ability in performance.

An example is the following statements recorded in the progress notes: "Arthur sits and sorts beads and flowers for four-and-a-half out of five minutes with 100% accuracy, but doing it at erratic speeds" (Progress note, 1978). The only place in the records where the staff comment informally is in the day-to-day progress notes.

Other students have not moved as of yet in the scheduled reorganization which was supposed to happen in December and January, so the classroom situation in regards to overloading has not improved. As a result, we are trying to keep Darryl in the program, but since he is over age for the Children's Department, he does not receive the full attention I believe his program deserves – there are other students under twenty-two years old in the program who require consideration. I anticipate having more time to spend with Darryl once the reorganization is complete. Darryl, in terms of progress, has joined in peer group activities, improved in fine motor task. However, progress has been somewhat inconsistent due to lack of time and staff. I feel next month's report, which will detail progression [in regard to] April evaluations should be more detailed. (Teacher, 1978)

Celia's toileting is no longer a priority because nineteen people in Apartment N were prioritized for toileting. The staff ratio is too low to toilet that many people. Also, toilets have not been adapted and Celia has no experience in toileting. She may be reprioritized in the future if the situation permits. (Psychologist, 1979)

Russel is considered unsuitable for a school program due to the difficulty of getting him in and out of the wheelchair and his inability to eat bag lunches. (Progress notes, 1978)

Decisions regarding transfer, implementation of a resident's program, or participation in school programs are determined not only by residents' needs but also by availability of the staff, progress to date, age, over-crowding, and the availability of appropriate equipment.

Although writing progress notes gradually becomes a requirement of the job, attendants comment reluctantly. Comments are optimistic, telling little of complications with residents or conditions in the environment. They often reveal a personal side of the resident not found in other records. The notes on Kerry over a seven-month period are indicative of actual notes written by different attendants.

February, 1978
"Kerry had a good evening." (Supervisor Attendant, A.M.)
"Kerry ate well today and seem[s] to have a good day." (Attendant 1)
"Kerry ate well and was a good boy all P.M." (Supervisor, P.M.)

March, 1978
"Kerry chewed his shirt sleeve again this p.m. Pulled P.J's off night stand, thought it was a huge joke." (Attendant 1)

"Kerry ate a good breakfast on feeding program at lunch. Really liked to play with his new musical T.V. box. As it played, he pointed to the moving scenes. When the music stopped, he started yelling (FOR MORE!)." (Attendant 2)

"Kerry was fresh today. He wiggled himself into M's (Apartment) clothing room and closed the door. When we found him, he laughed, like he thought it was a huge joke and that he had put something over on us." (Attendant 1)

August, 1978
"Kerry went over to the evaluation center today for a consultation with various doctors and nurses. They wanted to see what Kerry was capable of and what was voluntary and involuntary." (Attendant 2)

The notes written by attendants include specific circumstances which are increasingly revealing about the personality of the resident. Identifying a rationale for Kerry's laughter, for example, and interpreting the situation, the attendant describes volitional acts.

The following professional note in the record reveals the difference between the two descriptions. "Kerry made slight gains towards meeting his quarterly objective" (Music therapist, 1978). In another place, the objective from his Annual Review (1978–79) reads:

Annual Objective: When presented with a variety of musical activities, Kerry will participate by purposefully manipulating objects and pointing to directed body parts, and attending eye contact 50% of each activity. Quarterly Objective: Given the verbal clue to "touch his nose" in the context of an action song, Kerry will identify his nose three out of four times with physical assistance for three consecutive sessions. His resistance to assistance to touch his nose seems less. He has shown some improvement in peer interaction by some frequent eye contact also. The target date may be reset as this seems to be a realistic objective. Kerry will be included in leisure time music groups to be held once per week for one-half-hour on the ward. These will be implemented in August, conducted by staff music therapists with attendant assistance. (Music therapist, 1979)

In this note, what Kerry does is extraneous to what the professional tries to get the resident to do. For example, the teacher monitors the number of times per trial the resident performs the activity and the level of assistance necessary. The solution to questions of what to do with a resident and documentation of the progress made becomes the baseline data on performance and trials.

Throughout the entire review of records of 64 residents, only one set of formal reports refers to the residents as competent and capable of self-initiated action. The accident report identifies interaction of the residents with one another. The accident report lists seven possibilities for the accident or the injury in response to the question, "In your judgement, how did the accident occur?" (1) self caused by the resident, (2) caused during interaction between the residents, (3) caused by resident-to-resident assault, (4) occurred during interaction between staff person and resident, (5) resident self abusive, (6) other, (7) unknown and unexplained. Only item 2 formally attributes cause and effect to interaction between two residents. While these reports do not provide a detailed account of the circumstances surrounding the accidents, they do reveal the fact that residents do something on their own.

Twenty-eight accident reports mentioned scraps with another resident, sometimes with the same individual repeatedly. Beverly has a history of biting and scratching other residents, especially Danial. A series of notes confirms the resident-to-resident interaction which may be more than coincidental. The earliest note (August 1978) records that Danial was bitten twice. In December 1978, an aide spotted Beverly on the floor next to Danial, who was crying and pushing her away. From later reports, it appears that Beverly also hits Dennis, Gertrude, and Raymond. In the records of Danial and Beverly are a series of notes which indicate that when they are together, they are involved in biting and scratching. This culminates in a note by the building supervisor that Beverly and Danial are to be separated at all times.

> Beverly on mat in classroom. Beverly objects pulling Danial's hair. I went over to move Danial away from her so she wouldn't bother him any more and noticed the teeth marks where she bit him on his left forearm [Building director]. These two clients should be separated at all times. (Accident and injury report, 1979)

In December 1979, after the direction to keep the two residents apart, Beverly and Danial are at it again. What brings them together? That they are doing something is *as* significant as the fact that they have to be separated.

Supervision and control are not always deterrents. "Seth was standing near me when Margo came running. Seth had his hands up. Margo ran into him; Seth fell down and got a bump on his forehead, scratched on his head, and his lip bled" (Accident report, 1978).

Sometimes the same incident occurs over and over again. For instance, Janet turned herself over eight times in the course of 1978 and eventually was able to undo her straps and slide herself out, incurring abrasions and scratches in the process. For Christine, the process was noted as a deliberate act:

> LPN gives medication to another resident; I looked up just in time to see Christine twist her body with enough force to turn her wheelchair over with her seat belt buckled in place. Pulled at seat belt and it came unhooked and then she kicked the wheelchair away. (Accident report, 1978)

Sometimes staff develop a hypothesis to link events between the residents; "Gertrude on mat in classroom. Another girl was bothered by the fact that she was so close, so she scratched her left scapula and forearm" (Teacher, 1976). The attendants must prevent accidents from occurring. Otherwise they do not look for any significance in the interaction. In another example, the aide tells a resident helper to stop doing something. The resident inflicts his frustration on another resident for whom he is caring. "[Resident helper] slapped Maynard in the face because he was asked not to turn the beds around. As I turned around, he knocked the wheelchair over with Maynard in it" (Accident report, 1977). There are circumstantial accidents, as between May and Kim: "Kim had her head resting on May's leg. All of a sudden Kim lifted her head. When it came back down, she opened her mouth and bit May's leg just above the knee. Marks could be seen where Kim's teeth had been" (Accident report, 1978). The problem is to determine the circumstances that prompt the action – motive and intent, if any. Piecing together the story on the basis of the report, we are left to speculate about meaning.

Summary

Notes in residents' records (1975–81) are essentially a demonstration of the increasing sophistication of a program and its components: the case study, the annual review, and the individualized educational program. The case study method, the annual review, establishment of priorities for each resident within designated needs areas, accompanied by sophisticated techniques for the collection and analysis of behavior, on the whole provide a comprehensive picture of an individual's skills and abilities. Information is channelled through an increasingly uniform clinical system of collection and analysis of data.

The case study focuses on the individual. Nowhere in any case study is mention of another resident with whom the individual interacts, lives, eats, or attends school, except for the occasional accident report. Although social and personal dimensions are assessed, the assessment results are always in terms of the test and the examiner. The annual review incorporates program priorities. The plan for the program and the priorities are linear and additive – more needs, more programs, more resources and personnel. Development in priority areas means the increase or decrease in skills within need areas. The residents' achievements, their accomplishments, their growth and development are reduced to numerical values – the number of times performed, or the number of trials over a designated period of time. Not only are skills broken down and measured in this way, but behavior is controlled and managed similarly. Behaviors are broken down, counted, and timed as entities isolated from their relationship to the circumstances and events which surround them and out of which they develop.

Specialization and consultation further refine this systematic reduction and focus. Staff relate to one another within a disciplinary framework with its accompanying language and role system. Each presents a fragment of a whole, a clinical picture – not an overall view of the individual. Training attendants to record progress notes perpetuates the system and distances us from understanding what the residents actually *do*. The spontaneous reporting of events and interactions of residents with attendants – found infrequently in the early reports (that is, before 1975, when the Title XIX evaluations began) – almost totally disappears in progress notes written after 1975.

The reports paint a picture of each resident doing everything in isolation from the other residents with actions performed only when he or she interacts with staff. Notes of progress, examination descriptions, and records of objectives present no consistent picture of an individual's growth and development over the years of study, but rather reveal inconsistencies and contradictions. Confusion results from trying to distinguish whether or not the resident is withdrawn, unresponsive, passive to stimuli, or does not interact with his or her environment. Character traits are repeated in reports as if they were the more accurate statements about the resident. The jigsaw of impressions results from statements made in isolation from one another. Impressions gathered at a particular time and in a certain set of circumstances are recorded by a variety of individuals after any number of other interactions and events. Observations are not reported systematically. The following is one of the only statements in the records to mention "observation on the ward" (in addition to the therapist's three-page report on music ability):

Observation on the ward: In the apartment Melinda is often playing with and chewing on pieces of cloth or string. She has been observed walking around the apartment, sitting on the floor or mat and occasionally sleeping on her bed. When approached by staff, she often asks for a drink of water. (Music therapist, 1979)

Generally, observation is what precedes the lesson or intervention and is a means to determine where to begin, or what behavior to stop. Intervention accompanies the observation of behavior.

Non compliant during each month, missed school on occasion due to his erratic health status, spent a great deal of time in bed, was non-aggressive towards staff on occasions. I spent a lot of time observing him and interpreting his abnormal behavior by redirection to appropriate activities, reinforcing him when appropriate and giving him a chance to walk (inside and outside, which he enjoys very much). (Psychologist, 1980)

The poverty of our knowledge results from a limited focus on the immediate situation and literal translations of behavior. An example is the belief that communication is synonymous with speech – that if a resident doesn't speak, he doesn't communicate: "Severely and profoundly mentally retarded, blind, involuntary movements of upper and lower extremities and some spasticity. At the present time, he doesn't communicate; does not understand the spoken word" (Orthopedic note, 1973). The audiologist talks about another dimension, but makes the same point: "No constant response noted in speech, warble tones with narrow boundaries" (1980). Communication in this way is defined within the set boundaries of one dimension and one modality.

Russel indicated pleasure by vocalizing, laughing, and smiling when people were around him. No verbalizations nor sign language was observed. However, as Russel is handicapped by his physical limitations, neither model of communication was likely. Russel did not spontaneously point to the pictures on his board, but he did indicate a desire for people by reaching for them. (Speech and hearing department, 1978)

Summary

Although Russel indicates something in his actions, his *evaluation* on speech and communication is negligible. The teacher may not be able to distinguish if behavior is pathological, a seizure, or is something the resident decides to do. "Displaying a strange behavior, shaking his head and arms very hard in a quivering type way. We are not sure if it's a seizure or not. It may be self-induced behavior" (Teacher, 1978). Who the residents are and what they do, based on clinical knowledge, objectifies the individual as a behavior – an entity evaluated according to a norm or a standard. The residents are considered passive, helpless, in need of total care. The reports do not speak of the residents as active autonomous individuals who interact and "do things" on their own. The procedures for gathering and collecting information as well as the interpretation of the information are funnelled into a system of clinical facts.

Throughout the period of the study, development of programs for residents brought increased attention to the conduct of the programs themselves. The examination, the assessment, the establishment of priority skill areas for conduct of lessons and therapy sessions, and a scheme for behavior management all underlined a commitment to the program. In 1980, the residents were both subject and object of increased professional involvement and their structured existence was a far cry from the chaos of the custodial ward described by Fernald (1896).

Notes

1 The descriptive terms for the mentally handicapped in the "historical context" section of each chapter are those of the period. They illustrate the evolution of the references to the severely and the profoundly mentally handicapped and multiply handicapped.

2 Descriptions from the fieldnotes are set off from the text.

2

The perspective of the residents

In the name of humanity, then, in the name of modesty, in the name of wisdom, I intreat you to *place yourselves in the position* of those whose sufferings I describe, before you attempt to discuss what course is to be pursued towards them. Feel for them; try to defend them. Be their friends, – argue not hostilely. Feeling the ignorance to be in one sense real, which all of you confess on your lips, listen to one who can instruct you. Bring the ears and the minds of children, children as you are, or pretend to be, in knowledge – not believing without questioning, but questioning that you may believe. (*Perceval's Narrative: A Patient's Account of His Psychosis 1830–2*, Bateson, 1974:4; emphasis added)

The historical context

Our understanding and characterization of self and others change with increased knowledge. Our beliefs, attitudes, misconceptions, and prejudices about the mentally retarded are shaped by how we have gone about inquiry. The clinical model of interpretation, the herald of numerous significant advances in the identification and amelioration of pathology, is here described as the basis for understanding and interpretation of the functional aspects of ability.

The clinical gaze of medicine focuses on the relationship between the characteristics of disease and symptoms exhibited by the organism. The influence of positivism, which characterized scientific thought at the dawn of the nineteenth century in Paris, led to the conviction that a line could be drawn between normal and deviant organs based on the manifestation of etiological symptoms. This conviction and its inherent assumptions persist to the present.

Nineteenth century medicine ... was regulated more in accordance with normality than with health; it formed its concepts and prescribed its interventions in relation to a standard of functioning and organic structure, and physiological knowledge ... as [a] model ... these concepts were arranged in a space whose profound structure responded to the healthy morbid opposition. When one spoke of the life of groups and societies, of the life of the race, or even of the "psychological life," one did not think first of the internal structure of *the organized being* but of *the medical bipolarity of the normal and the pathological.* (Foucault, 1975:35)

54

Positivism entailed a faith that the medical observer could make a rational connection between the diverse characteristics observed in the organs of the patient and the description of disease.

Within the clinical model, difference is defined as deviation and irregularity from an idealized, normative conception of the human condition and functioning. The organs of the body perform specific functions. Since the presence or absence of particular functions is associated with impairment to the organs, *cause and effect* of the pathology are sought in the *organic* features of the organism. A pathological system is a set of biological symptoms observed in the body which hinders, impedes, or changes normal processes and functioning. A syndrome category classifies the symptoms observed, and is rated for closeness of fit to the description provided for each syndrome category in the typology of medical syndromes. The prognosis changes as the disease develops in the organism. The treatment is modified to suit changes in the course of the disease until normal functioning is restored.

An assumption of the model is that normality versus pathology is a dichotomy. Can complex human systems be explained by this duality? The answer from the perspective of the clinical model is to determine the degree and the range of difference in the organic systems of the individual. Judgement within this framework is *unidirectional*, a clinical decision that supports the hypothesis of deviancy as distinct from normal functioning. The observer focuses on the identification of pathology by determining differences, then syndromes. In the process of observation the clinician matches the symptoms with the description of known diseases and pathologies. Then the description contained in the categories for a syndrome determines what the clinician looks for. The process of matching is *categorical*.

Medical typologies are standard *universal* descriptions of disease. A highly specialized body of knowledge about disease and pathology develops as a set of facts. The factual description of disease and pathology evolves within the typology; similar cases map boundaries to a disease and the range of variation and make general statements about prognosis and treatment. The formalized categories and associations to which the clinical observer refers in the typology in turn reinforce the ability to distinguish the pathological from the normal.

Underlying the historical, social, political, and economic developments in the care of the mentally retarded is the notion of an ideal person, a standard for comparison, and of cultural and societal norms of appearance and behavior (Rhodes and Head, 1974:36).

The severely and profoundly mentally retarded and multiply handicapped form a remarkable, heterogeneous group of individuals, the antithesis of the ideal type and at variance with functioning within the social order.

The perspective of the residents

Since their ability is determined in clinical terms and the clinical terms dictate a certain type of care, the position of the severely handicapped remains outside the mainstream of society. Clinical descriptions and psychological and educational evaluations provide only a partial description of who they are.

Aspects of the clinical model of interpretation referred to in current literature on the mentally retarded are the pathological, statistical, and cultural differences. Mercer describes the pathological and statistical models as derivatives of the clinical perspective.

The clinical perspective classifies the mentally retarded as a handicapping condition, which exists in the individual and can be diagnosed by clinically trained professionals using properly standardized assessment techniques...

The clinical perspective is the frame of reference commonly adopted by persons in the helping professions – those in the field of medicine, psychology, social work, and education. Within this general perspective, there are two contrasting definitions of "normal": the pathological model contributed by medicine and the statistical model advanced by psychology and education. The two approaches are used interchangeably by clinicians...

The pathological model of normal was developed in medicine as a conceptual tool for comprehending and controlling disease processes and organic malfunctioning. Medical concern is aroused when conditions occur which interfere with the physiological functions of the organism. Consequently the focus of the medical model is on pathology and the symptoms of pathology. Diseases are defined by the biological symptoms which characterize them. Emphasis is on defining the nature of the abnormal, and normal tends to be treated as a residual category containing organisms that do not have abnormal symptoms; abnormal = presence of pathological symptoms...

[The statistical model] defines abnormality according to the extent to which an individual varies from the average of the population on a particular trait...

In establishing norms, the investigator uses the characteristics of the particular population being studied to establish the boundaries of normal. Unlike the bipolar pathological model, the statistical model defines two types of abnormals: those who have abnormally large amounts of the characteristic measured and those who have abnormally small amounts. (Mercer, 1973:2–4)

Each of these models supports the prejudicial stereotype of the underlying and pervasive paradigm of "handicapism." "We define it as a set of assumptions and practices that promote the differential and unequal treatment of people because of apparent or assumed physical, mental, or behavioral differences" (Bogdan and Biklen, 1977:14). The individual is the *object* of the study but not the *subject* acting. The whole of the individual becomes a diagnostic picture, a constellation of objective clinical facts.

Having established the clinical definition of pathological characteristics, the individual assumes a position relative to the mainstream in society – that is, the relationship of the severely and profoundly mentally retarded and multiply handicapped to society is built from a definition of their pathology established through clinical processes. The numerical norms of the statistical model rest on the comparison of the severely and profoundly mentally retarded and multiply handicapped with the normal population. Debates over the methods of the statistical model in establishing the norms do not change the fundamental nature of the comparison. The focus on the basic differences of the severely and profoundly mentally retarded and multiply handicapped calls into question both the comparison and the methods.

The reality of disability is a cultural definition of the disabled at variance with a society or culture's mainstream norms and expectations for behavior. The cultural model, essentially a restatement of the clinical model, emphasizes their difference. The concept of culture is the criterion that makes the mentally retarded a subgroup of the society. For example, Lewis (1933) proposed one distinction between pathological and subcultural types of mental retardation. A subcultural type refers to a cultural deviation from the norm or a cultural deficiency determined by variation within that culture: in other words, such an individual belongs to the lower end of the normal distribution. By contrast a pathological definition of the severely and profoundly retarded refers to manifest organic differences which disallow any cultural application. According to Lewis's distinction, the severely and profoundly mentally retarded do not even attain subcultural status because of the conglomeration of their pathological manifestations.

Current references to the mentally retarded as a subhuman, deviant subgroup, subcultural, acultural, culturally deviant, and culturally marginal, do not parallel Lewis's cultural distinction but convey a similar pejorative quality.

A presumably subhuman individual is usually perceived as being potentially assaultive, destructive, and lacking in self-direction and constructive purposes; this necessitates restricting his movements both to control him more easily, and to protect either the human from the subhuman or one subhuman from another...

Subhumans are either not expected to learn or develop appreciably, or their growth potential is seen as so small as to be irrelevant, since it will never lead to complete humanization. In other words the state of sub-humanity is perceived as being essentially permanent, or at least to last as long as the person resides in the building [within an institution]. In consequence, the environment may be designed to maintain a client's level of functioning at best, but not necessarily to provide opportunities for further growth and development. (Wolfensberger, 1972:63–66)

Such a construction rests on the idea of "man-as-trivium," a human being who is not to be taken seriously or given importance. (Wolfensberger, 1972:68, citing Vail, 1967)

The perspective of the residents

The severely and profoundly mentally retarded are seen as a subpopulation who do not fully share a common human capacity with the dominant culture. They have no common ground. By social contract, the population occupies a position below or outside of the society, devalued, close to an animal or vegetable state, belittled, aberrant, without human qualities.

This system of beliefs which regards the retarded as a menace, suffering, holy innocent, a diseased organism, object of ridicule, or an eternal child perpetuates the cultural bias within clinical classifications (Wolfensberger, 1972, 1975). Ethnocentric beliefs, attitudes, and values perpetuate and provide the justification for the nature of their treatment and the maintenance of their social position.

These conceptualizations of the mentally retarded are grounded, not in understanding them in their own terms, but rather in our beliefs and attitudes. Consequently the education and care of the mentally retarded depend on their socialization from the institution into the mainstream of society. In turn, treatment services to rehabilitate the individual impose criteria of performance and at the same time define expected ability. Movement into the mainstream becomes a linear ascension of skill acquisition (Reynolds 1967). The ladder of ability becomes a subtle set of standards based on the same assumptions as the clinical diagnosis. Remedies are suggested at the level of alternatives to existing institutional models, or the realignment of the residents within mainstream society. Seldom do we question the basis of inquiry or the type of knowledge on which we base our understanding and make decisions.

The institution itself does not mirror or demonstrate normal living and working conditions nor, more significantly, normal interactions. The residents in institutions must learn twice: to interpret the communications of the other residents and care providers, and to handle interactions in other environments and settings in the mainstream. They must demonstrate competence in socialization in the institution to gain participation outside of the institution and assimilation into the community. For example, Edgerton (1967) studied the mildly mentally retarded to see how they managed their lives after hospitalization and the reintroduction to mainstream culture. He documented the existence of private and public images in which they deny the reality of their retardation in order to pass into the mainstream culture. Their denial illustrates the cultural dissonance they experience.

Two current studies differentiated cultural deviance of the severely mentally retarded by studying the population in mainstream cultural terms. Wills (1971, 1973), like Lewis, drew cultural distinctions among the severely mentally retarded living on wards within an institution. In his 1971 study, he differentiated the "more" and "less" capable residents based on mainstream cultural expectations of ability. In his 1973 study, this distinction was further refined to "cultural" and "acultural." The latter study differentiated among residents based on mainstream cultural categories: for example, sitting and watching television is a cultural behavior by which the degree of their mainstream ability is determined.

The distinction between culture and nonculture used here refers to the presence or absence of behavior which is uniquely human. It does not refer to the ability to behave according to the norms of a particular human society. The researcher did not conduct the study with this twofold distinction in mind. Instead the distinction was recognized only after observations were collected, categories had been formulated, and observations were coded in terms of the categories. (Wills, 1973:5)

A review of cultural references in the literature on mental retardation reveals that the notion of culture is used to delineate differences between the mainstream culture and the retarded (MacAndrew and Edgerton, 1964; Wills, 1973; Landesman-Dwyer, 1974). In these studies, the researcher translates and interprets the mentally retarded experience in mainstream terms, categories, and meanings (not in their *own* terms) to understand the difference in their experience.

A cultural investigation cannot be a rewording of the conventional and traditional understandings which characterize the severely and profoundly mentally retarded as separate and apart from the mainstream, or describe and compare them against cultural norms of performance. The behavior of the severely and profoundly mentally retarded can only be defined in categories and terms which match their experience. A cultural interpretation proceeds from standards, characteristics, categories, and definitions emerging from their unique life circumstances on mats and in cribs. Mainstream cultural criteria are artificial, in that their application confuses and glosses over the significance and meaning of their differences. Without fundamental awareness grounded in observation of their conduct of daily life, any cultural interpretation of the severely and profoundly mentally retarded and multiply handicapped is tied to clinical assumptions.

Goffman's *Asylums* (1961) details those processes which maintain institutionalization and challenges those settings which stigmatize the individual. Institutionalization maintains cultural isolation (Goffman, 1963, 1967). It is segregation from society which then becomes the focus of public attention and which current efforts to reintegrate the disabled population are attempting to rectify. This shift in setting is not, however, a fundamental shift in perspective and understanding of the disabled. Rather it is a recognition of basic rights and recognition of past shortcomings and inequities.

Blatt's (1970, 1973; Blatt and Kaplan, 1974) popular exposés of institutional life in words and pictures focuses attention on conditions within the institution.

What attendants say and do continues the stereotype of the residents, institutions and programs (Bogdan and Taylor 1974, 1975). The literature reporting what attendants say and do assumes deviancy and focuses on institutional life from the standpoint of what is done to the residents rather than what the residents do. While understanding of the institution is fundamental to understanding what we, the professionals do, it may *not* be as fundamental to understanding what the residents do beyond clarifying the constraints within which they function.

The individual

Within the literature of first-person accounts on the disabled is a consistent theme – the recognition by family members and care givers of unique patterns and qualities in interactions with the severely and profoundly mentally retarded and multiply handicapped. Beyond the clinical definition of the condition emerges a recognition of communicative patterns. Bogdan and Taylor (1982) challenge the meaning of mental retardation as a clinical designation with first person accounts of the mentally retarded residents of an institution. They argue for acceptance of the mentally retarded persons outside the conceptions of the label.

First person accounts of the handicapped, specifically the mentally retarded, are usually written by parents and family members (see Murray 1967; Buck 1950; Anderson 1963; Deacon 1974; Greenfield 1965, 1978; Higgins 1970; Kaufman 1980; Roberts and Roberts 1962; Turner 1980). Others are by educators (Bancroft 1915) and superintendents of training schools (Johnstone 1923). These stories, ostensibly about the mentally retarded and the handicapped in different contexts – home, school, and institution – are written from the perspective of the parent, teacher, or superintendent. The accounts are parental pictures of family life, the fears, worries and trials of finding help, teacher accounts of frustration and the patience required to teach a child to perform a task, and descriptions of life at the institution. Each account tries to recreate the story of the handicapped persons themselves but never in their own words.

One account is different, *The World of Nigel Hunt: The Diary of a Mongoloid Youth* (1967). Nigel tells his story in his own words. He learned to read and type and recorded the diary of his experiences and travels.

My mother has been so kind to me all my life. My mother taught me to read. When I was very tiny we used to play together with plastic letters and a book with huge letters on it. I learned the sounds of the letters from my mother as we played.
After I had learned the sound of every letter, mother held things up and

sound-spelled them like, "This is a C U P" and soon I could do it all by myself; all our friends were amazed and pleased with me when I began to read properly from books. (Hunt, 1967:97–98)

In the foreword, Dr. Penrose acknowledges the significance of an account of the world as Nigel sees it. Nigel's experience is significant but Penrose uses the data to characterize Nigel's retardation. He is described as possessing the classical features and temperament of the anomaly: preoccupation with musical performance, friendliness and a rich sense of humor, and the concrete manner of his thinking, found in his observations and descriptions (Hunt, 1967:9–13).

In considering the severely and profoundly mentally retarded and multiply handicapped, it is precisely the multiple and divergent nature of their expression which does not invite generalization. As the multiple nature of her son's disability becomes clearer, Featherstone (1981), like Penrose, identifies the way in which the patterns of the disability are her initial focus.

Amid the storm of emotions surrounding the Featherstone family's growing awareness of Jodi's multiple disabilities and their individual and collective journeys towards understanding and acceptance of Jodi's difference, Featherstone (1981) reflects that if the family were not coping with Jodi's disability "our other problems would expand to fill the void. With this realization I began to look at Jodi's disabilities a little differently. They became part of the pattern of my life rather than the dominant motif" (p. 221).

At this point in her thinking, Jodi was the disability. Even parents intimately familiar with their child talk about the disability as being the central focus of their experience. The change in perception is from understanding Jodi's disability to understanding Jodi.

When Jodi was fifteen months old we learned that he was blind. We wept for the experiences he would miss. Yet we realized how much remained – if he were only blind. Most of the activities that gave our lives meaning and importance would still be within his reach. He could read, write, teach, play, and enjoy the fellowship of friends. He could talk and think, give comfort and, in time, go about his own life independently, perhaps with some special understanding born of his disability. Anyway, that is what we hoped. The idea of blindness made us sad. It led us to examine our values: it did not shatter them. However, as the months went by we learned that Jodi was not only blind. He had cerebral palsy; he was probably severely retarded. During the first eighteen months of his life he cried almost continually from pain that no one could diagnose or relieve. His days and nights were passed in misery; his future looked bleak and limited. Hardly a day passed without our asking ourselves whether his life was worth living. Each of us, separately and together, wished for an end to his ordeal: a peaceful, painless death.

He did not die. He was remarkably tough. Unexpectedly, after the doctors removed an infected shunt, his pain went. He cried less during the day and slept longer at night. He smiled more often, even laughed. Liberated from his inner torments he responded to us. We began to like him. He gave more; his smiles, his laughter, his delighted shrieks. He asked less. He still needed a lot of special care, but we no longer performed our family routines with one hand while patting a wretched baby with the other. Each of us began to feel that Jodi's life was worth living, and that he made his own special contribution to the family.

Barring a miracle, Jodi will not lead a "useful independent life." He will not read and write; he may never talk to friends in the way that we do. He will always depend on others for his basic needs. Yet he maintains a vital human connection to the people and events around him. He is part of a web of shared experience. He makes us aware of our own fragility and limitations, and of how much we share with people whose interests and circumstances differ dramatically from our own. He contributes in his own quiet way. (Featherstone, 1981:235–236)

The parental pain at the loss of unfilled dreams and expectations for their child that comes with the identification of blindness, cerebral palsy, and mental retardation is a pain that at first seems capable of alleviation only by "a peaceful, painless death." Gradually, however, a second and more profound realization is made of the experience. What can Jodi do? Jodi is "remarkably tough" he smiles and *even* laughs. Jodi responds to us: "We began to like him. He *gave more*; his smiles, his laughter, his *delighted shrieks*. He *asked less*" (my emphasis). In his own quiet ways he maintains "a vital human connection to people and events around him." What experience does he share? How did he give more and ask less? What is the meaning of his delighted shrieks?

Gradually over time there emerges a pattern to what Jodi does. In acceptance of the disability, Featherstone moves on to the identification of the patterns in Jodi's behavior and redefinition of his experience. Featherstone comes to see beyond Jodi's disability to identify the experiences that Jodi shares with us. What he contributes demonstrates his connection to a shared common experience. In realizing Jodi's ability, Featherstone accepts that Jodi will not lead a "useful independent life" in the ways she would have defined it previously. Understanding begins with a reconceptualization of the effect of the handicap on the person.

It is asymmetries in interpretation of the disability that give rise to misunderstandings of who the disabled are. This asymmetry comes from a misplaced and disproportionate emphasis on the disability. A balanced interpretation of their ability can emerge from a consideration of their ability in context. Their performance is related to the characteristics of their condition and pathology as well as to the other dimensions of human experience. Programs and interventions which focus on attributes of pathology miss essential elements of the interaction and participation in what the residents are doing. A specialist who observes the residents' behavior in this setting can apply a clinical form of inquiry to support an interpretation of disability. Specialized analysis by doctors, educators, therapists, and psychologists may fragment interpretation of behavior because of the way information is gathered. Each discipline contributes a part of the whole; assessment and subsequent intervention develop in each case from an isolated focus on specific skills. A picture of the whole, of what the individual can actually do, never seems to coalesce. This occurs for various reasons. Intention and purposeful behavior are not even considered; information gained from each separate focus is not integrated; mastery and proficiency displayed by each resident in daily life are minimally considered. In this way, competence is not considered and context is ignored.

Clinical forms of inquiry which categorize behaviors as symptoms of a central nervous system disorder predominate with this population. Establishing a framework for interpretation involves searching for the correspondence between underlying organic causes and behavior as characteristic of a particular classification, such as blind, deaf, or mentally retarded. A clinical portrait of each individual develops as a list of problems which each individual manifests. This clinical description stereotypes the residents, and makes assumptions about what care and treatment ought to be.

A focus on pathology cuts short any further exploration of an individual's unique ability to cope and adapt within his or her life circumstances. Within any broad handicapping classification, individual behavior or ability is studied as a separate entity – for example information processing, language ability, or eye tracking. A particular ability is studied, not within the framework of an integrated understanding of the individual's functioning, but as an isolated characteristic of a handicapping condition. For instance, the severely and profoundly mentally retarded and multiply handicapped have different motor abilities, but may also possess will and determination adequate to explore movement within their constraints – although neither is a general characteristic of their disability.

Interpretations based on the presence or absence of a particular skill or process short-circuit a view of purposeful behavior. Information obtained through the systematic use of behavioral scales and indices does not challenge the categories used. Behaviors are judged, rated, and recorded for closeness of fit to the prescribed category. When fitting an observed repertoire into a behavioral category – for example, watching television or sitting – the mainstream standard of performance is the expectation by which performance is judged. The same organic differences by which they were categorized at the time of institutionalization are now assumed to be modifiable to mainstream standards and conventions, even though there is no substantially new understanding or clarification of the organic systems to justify such a shift. Recognition of which behaviors can be modified and which are stable and enduring frustrates and challenges educational and rehabilitative efforts.

This frustration is rarely resolved and creates a constant tension in the conduct of practice. One result is the stylized interaction by staff. Communication with the residents becomes a series of predetermined commands and reinforcements. Secondly, an intervention once adopted is adhered to rigorously, despite limited progress towards the criteria set. Thirdly, the proliferation of behavioral objectives across all areas of functioning is a self-perpetuating system by which practice is directed. Fourthly, revision of practice often reflects the fluctuating trends and concepts within a discipline without careful examination of the assumptions on which those trends are based or integral knowledge of the individual. Finally, behavior modification, assumed to be one of the only techniques appropriate for this population, neglects a fuller analysis of behavior in context; the concentration on specific behavioral change according to set criteria *precludes* a fuller description.

Example 1: Beverly and Jamie

In the following description, a psychologist observes the behavior of two residents, Jamie and Beverly. The psychologist drops his formal method of observation with Beverly to become absorbed in the naturally occurring events with Jamie. Such differences in observation may account in part for the varied interpretations of the residents' ability in the records. The clinical description, while necessary for understanding various features of Jamie's handicapping condition, pales in light of her ability to work within the restrictions of the handicap.

The psychologist demonstrates the ability to switch modes of observation, understanding, and involvement with the residents. His involvement with Jamie is different from his involvement with Beverly. He comments on different attributes of Jamie's behavior and involves himself in her struggle for freedom. By contrast, he directs and controls Beverly's behavior. In the parallel descriptions of Jamie and Beverly, a different picture emerges from between the lines.

On this particular morning, some residents were not in school due to a cancellation of their regular classes.

After the meal cart was rolled out of that portion of the activity room used as the dining area, and after all the teachers, therapists, and nurses picked up and transported to various rooms up and down the corridor most of the residents, I observed the following events. Jamie and five other residents were not taken to school. In the middle of a pathway through the mats on the floor, Jamie and three others were seated in their wheelchairs. I focused my attention on Jamie as I observed her hand fingering the spokes of her right wheel.

Jamie was slumped over in her chair with her head bowed to the right. Her pupils were barely visible through her drooping eyelids. Eye contact was impossible. How was Jamie going to spend her morning on the ward? The time was 9:45.

While I was watching Jamie, the psychologist for the ward entered slowly pushing Beverly in a wheelchair. As he leaned over Beverly's head he held her hands down onto the wheels of the chair attempting to teach her to wheel the chair. She slouched, compressed from the encompassing hug. When released, Beverly's hand flailed up against the side of her head and she bit the knuckle of her thumb, repeating this sequence over and over, faster and faster. Repeating the command, "Hands down!" the psychologist removed Beverly from the chair and put her on the mat. He took a stopwatch from around her neck and a clipboard out of the pouch on the back of her chair and started to measure the frequency and the length of time between Beverly's hand motions. This time sample of behavior was recorded later on graphs to indicate the increase or decrease of hitting behavior after this activity. This was the standard means to record behavior.

Beverly's hitting behavior is regarded as a symptom of a central nervous system disorder and therefore, inappropriate. The procedure established to record the behavior isolates it as a unit to be counted. The assumption that the central nervous system is the cause for the behavior prevents a more complete understanding of the meaning in the action.

For instance, I had observed Beverly initiate this behavior when staff tried to get her to do something she did not want to do. The behavior at times is a signal to convey her frustration at being disrupted, not a behavior caused by a central nervous system disorder. The context for its occurrence provides this necessary clue. This information was not available unless her behavior was observed continuously and systematically over a long time in a variety of situations and activities with different people.

The psychologist sat observing Beverly on the mat. When an aide asked what he was doing, he remarked, "Watching specific behaviors when the residents are trying to do something." The stopwatch clicked; the behavior was recorded on a frequency-over-time graph until the hitting stopped.

On several occasions the psychologist had asked me, "What are you doing?" I had replied, "I am watching the actions of the residents."

That morning he asked, "So you want to see what everyone does? Well, here it's all medical and biological, not psychological. This is mental retardation versus mental health." "Oh," I said, "What is mental health?" He replied, "Psychosocial, where you can talk to the patients. Here you have to get all from behavior. It's all mixed up. What they are and what they eat is all together. Yes, observation can be interesting."

These statements reveal his underlying assumptions about Beverly and other residents. Beverly's handicaps are so severe that psychological processes revealing intent and purpose are dismissed. Further, because she cannot talk, it is assumed there is no possibility of confirmation by communication or interaction. Behavior is the only avenue to understand Beverly and the way to understand it is to count it.

Observing Beverly's behavior, the psychologist attends to and counts one unit of behavior. In concentrating on one behavior, he loses any message contained in Beverly's hitting herself. Other body movements and her reactions to what was happening are not related. Comparisons between this situation and others are not drawn. In this instance, interpretation and explanation are restricted and directed to the behavior being counted. The methodology isolates the attention of the observer, directing it away from a search for alternative interpretations and the application of a fuller contextual understanding. The knowledge generated in this system is self-perpetuating. The results recorded provide no new insight or challenge to the assumptions and knowledge on which they are based.

At 10:15, while the psychologist continued to record Beverly's hitting, Jamie, in slow deliberate pushes, pulls, and tugs on the wheel of her chair, bumped other chairs and mats covering the floor, and sandwiched herself between the wheelchairs and mats. The psychologist turned his attention to Jamie and commented, "Jamie, you got to be careful, separate, and lift up." (He was telling her how to unlock her chair.) She freed her chair and headed out the door. The psychologist laughed, "Freedom! All right! Go!" A sentiment was attributed to her actions.

An attendant glanced over and yelled, "Jamie's out the door!" No one moved. A nurse's aide returned her twenty minutes later saying, "O.K., you guys, Jamie was almost out the front door." (This was impossible because a fire door separated the corridor from the main hallway and the front doors.) The aide wheeled her into the circle again and departed. The psychologist interrupted marking his graph and said, "Next time, Jamie, take your coat." The aide left shutting the door. The psychologist addressed Jamie on the basis of purpose in her action.

Ten minutes later, Jamie turned her chair away from the group and wheeled herself out the other door. No one noticed her departure. In two minutes, she was returned by an attendant from another ward, who exclaimed, "Jamie was down the hall." She wheeled her into the center of the room again and departed, blocking the second entrance to the corridor. The psychologist went up to Jamie and spoke into her ear, "All the doors are shut to you. What are you going to do now?" He pointed to the door into the sleeping area. Jamie looked and started to go. At this point, not only did the psychologist identify purpose and intent but also began active participation in her endeavor.

As she inched toward the door, the supervisor for the ward caught her and turned her around as he said, "Where are you going?" He wheeled her into the circle and walked on. The fourth time she maneuvered out of the circle, Jamie caught her chair on the edge of the mat. Now totally absorbed in these episodes, the psychologist said, "O.K., roadblock." He got up and lifted her chair over the mat. Having identified with Jamie's struggle, the psychologist provided reassurance and help.

Meanwhile, the custodian rolled in a bucket and mop to wash that section of the floor used as the dining area. Jamie started across the floor; he grabbed the chair and pushed her back from where she came. He pulled a table across her pathway. Seeing this, the psychologist said to Jamie, "Don't worry, my money is with you." The psychologist was willing to wager more than assurances. After the floor dried, and the table was returned to its proper place, Jamie immediately darted out again. The psychologist said, "Where you off to?" Surprised, he questioned her intent, which was not immediately evident. The custodian stared at her, grabbed her chair again, and pushed her back. He then used the table as a barrier. The psychologist stated, "You're doing fine." Having offered this reassurance, he collected his clipboard and left the room. He did not continue his involvement with Jamie nor make further note of Beverly's behavior.

Jamie sat for five minutes swinging her head back and forth. After this pause, she went around the table and the divider for this area into the office. She was wheeled out by a primary caretaker. Jamie immediately turned her wheelchair and returned to the office. Since no one was there, she stayed for twenty minutes. With head bowed, she flipped through a magazine.

In observing Jamie, the psychologist makes a shift in both the method of observation and the nature of participation. Observation is focused on Jamie's demonstrated competency in the evolving circumstances in which she finds herself, rather than attention being directed to a specific behavior or skill.

In turning his attention to Jamie outside of the system for recording behavior, the psychologist allowed himself to move through successive stages of seeing, knowing, participating and empathy with what Jamie was up to. He began by telling her what to do; secondly, he attributed sentiment; thirdly, he acknowledged purpose in her actions, fourthly, he identified intent and ability; fifthly, he provided assurance and help and, finally, he participated. In so doing, the psychologist identified something similar and familiar in Jamie's actions. He identified intent, purpose, and a pattern in her behavior. The unit of analysis is not an individual's ability, such as hitting behavior, or wheeling a wheelchair, but rather the manifestation of an entire range of ability identifiable through attention to context. Competence in this instance becomes the demonstrated mastery and proficiency with which she accomplishes her tasks. The psychologist's participation changes to active involvement and collaboration in what she is up to.

Because similar assumptions underlie his participation with Jamie and with Beverly, he was surprised each time Jamie was returned. The psychologist's comments attributed human qualities to Jamie's actions, but his engagement with her was only secondary to what he was already doing. He did not follow the entire sequence closely, nor did he stay to see her achieve her goal, which dramatized her determination, persistence, and purpose.

Duty calls, the time for observing Beverly is up, therefore participation with Jamie is over. In not following the entire sequence, the psychologist overlooks an opportunity to understand more completely what Jamie does. Even with an appreciation of the obstacles she has encountered and overcome, he does not understand that the entire activity was initiated by Jamie to achieve a goal. No record of her achievement was made. No record of this event nor of Jamie's performance is made. No behavioral objective for Jamie is modified. Not even an anecdotal comment appears in the daily progress notes. In the end, he had not taken Jamie seriously. The psychologist does not realize the significance of the switch he has made in his method of observation and in his participation. Consequently he does not reflect on the difference in his observation and involvement with Jamie to what he is doing with Beverly.

The objective method of counting behaviors with Beverly is limited to the relative time the psychologist has to observe. Antecedent events are not taken into consideration. The focus is predetermined by an identified problem; when hitting behavior stops, the observation stops; subsequent behavioral sequences are not related to what is observed. Comparison of behaviors across contexts is not possible with the data collected in this way.

The residents express messages through the persistent repetition of behaviors. Such patterns develop in spite of their physical and neurological handicaps. Observation within a system for recording behavior is not enough. Following interesting events and chance encounters can be just as superficial as the search for correspondence between medical, psychological, and educational categories. Seeing without understanding is inadequate.

In her travels Jamie demonstrates a pattern of competence much more sophisticated than her skill assessment record. To wheel herself independently a distance of thirty feet is one example of a behavioral objective. The last recorded assessment of her skill level on this objective reads:

Jamie can independently wheel her chair ten feet. However, because of lack of motivation and noncompliant behavior she requires partial physical assistance while motivation is being established. (Education program objectives report, 1978)

Who can doubt Jamie's motivation in this event? The proficiency with which Jamie explores her environment is an evolving set of circumstances despite restrictions. First, Jamie demonstrates competence in assessing alternatives. She negotiates around obstacles, people, and things which thwart her goal. Her achievements surpass her performance in structured activities to meet the specific criteria of the behavioral objective. Secondly, Jamie expresses a message in the pattern of where she wants to go and what she wants to do. In her repetition of behaviors she demonstrates adaptive problem-solving competence. She is not taught problem solving ability as a skill but has learned it to accomplish what she wants. These patterns of competence develop despite her physical and neurological handicaps. Her persistence and determination to do what she wants provide evidence not only of a goal in mind but of a plan for its attainment. After a review of the situation, she acts, adjusting components of her routine, correcting for errors, and incorporating the assistance of the psychologist to achieve her goal. Jamie actively pursues and accomplishes her goal of getting out of the ward and into the office to flip the pages of a magazine.

The tension in what the psychologist does arises from the concentration of his prescribed interaction with Beverly, which he steps out of in his interaction with Jamie. His attention in counting the behavior of Beverly becomes participation with Jamie. With Beverly, he attempts to stop her hitting behavior; with Jamie, he is fascinated and becomes involved. The interpretations of Beverly's behavior and Jamie's endeavors could achieve greater symmetry if the professional's intervention complemented what the residents do.

The asymmetry reveals itself in the psychologist's interpretation of the two girls' behavior. On the one hand, he focused on keeping Beverly's hand down on the wheel of the wheelchair and counted the number of times that she hit herself; on the other hand, he attended to context and the meaning behind Jamie's efforts. However, he did not understand the significance of what he was doing. The differences in interpretation are not just differences in the observation, rather differences in knowing what lies at the heart of professional practice with the severely and profoundly mentally retarded and multiply handicapped.

The symmetric interpretation results from a broader consideration of the willful and intentional action of Jamie in the pursuit of a goal outside the constraints of her disability. Actually a symmetric interpretation results as the psychologist follows the meaning and the intention in her endeavors. He adopts her perspective.

Illusions of interpretation in professional practice

The asymmetry evident in the psychologist's interpretation of Jamie's and Beverly's behavior points to some fallacies of practice in this setting. These fallacies arise out of the ways in which we go about understanding the behavior of the severely and profoundly mentally retarded and multiply handicapped.

First is the fallacy of total reliance on clinical observation and description for understanding the residents. Knowledge of Jamie and Beverly is based exclusively on understanding behavior as a manifestation of organic systems and processes; the fact that Jamie was averbal, spastic, quadriplegic with cerebral palsy due to unknown causes and subject to central nervous system degeneration with an intelligence quotient under 20; and that Beverly's intelligence quotient was under 20, and that she was clinically blind, microcephalic, quadriplegic, spastic, and non-ambulatory only serve to highlight the significance of the event. Beverly activates her behavior as a signal of her distress at being made to wheel the wheelchair. Jamie accomplishes much more than can be understood by a listing of medical complications.

In the example, Beverly's and Jamie's communicative competence and purposeful action in events require a broader understanding and application of knowledge. A complete picture of who the residents are and what they do can only be gained by observation and description of how they function. Comparing different contexts in which Beverly activates hitting behavior provides a clue as to whether or not she hits herself as an act of defiance. Is the wheelchair activity an appropriate substitution for the self-abusive behavior if it, in turn, causes the self-abusive behavior?

The second fallacy is the assumption that Beverly's experience is directly translatable into educational skills and abilities. Jamie's and Beverly's actions can only be described in relation to the total context of events, the processes, and the routines used to communicate and achieve their goals. Fitting these processes and relations into the static categories, labels, and definitions found in the record does not capture their development, evolution or significance. Reduction of the individuals' experience to these categories limits our understanding of their competence and misrepresents what they actually do.

The third fallacy lies in the reduction of verbal communication with the residents to short, simple, repetitious commands such as "Hands down!" These declarative statements reflect the assumption that it is best to tell the residents what they are expected to do. Short quick commands may communicate an entirely different message to the resident.

The psychologist's comments to Jamie arise spontaneously out of interest in her actions and enthusiastic participation in wanting her to achieve her goal. The question by the psychologist, "Where you off to?" acknowledges her personal autonomy. The psychologist is delighted, offering her encouragement, pointing out options and experiencing satisfaction when the suggested route is tried. There is a different quality to this communication.

The fourth fallacy is that Beverly and Jamie's learning is governed by the stimulus-and-response reinforcement principles of learning theory, and that this is the most appropriate teaching methodology. Both Beverly and Jamie differentially discriminate contexts. They *read* the situations in which they find themselves. No single stimulus or reinforcement is evident. Jamie's getting out of the apartment and into the office despite all obstacles is inner-directed; she is motivated to do something. What that is does not become clear until the entire sequence of events evolves (over 95 minutes).

Observation of the context of the behavior achieves more than isolation of a probable stimulus. Observation illuminates the discrimination inherent in problem-solving in day-to-day life, in analysis of abilities in task performance, and in the activation of behavior repertoires over time.

From the earlier description emerges a picture of the patterns of Jamie's conduct of everyday life. When left on her own, she moves her wheelchair out of the apartment and around barriers repeatedly to find something of interest to her. Travels on her own exceed the documentation of her need for physical assistance or the notations in the record of being able to mobilize 10 feet, 30 feet, and 5 to 8 feet. The notations by the direct care staff of her "laughing and wheeling around merrily" (November 1979) come the closest to capturing some sense of her initiative and mobility. Further details as to what she actually did that afternoon are not recorded. Both the educational and therapeutic statements and the progress notes of the attendant do not capture her persistence and determination in the face of obstacles.

Beverly's structured wheelchair program is directed by the psychologist by commands, directives, and holding her hands down onto the wheels. What he sees is captured on the observational chart. It becomes the record of Beverly's performance in a structured programmed activity.

The description I have given reveals the dilemma posed for staff in interpretations of the resident's ability. The psychologist uses different information to interpret the behavior of the two residents. He is surprised by the contrasts between Jamie's expected and actual behavior. For example, with Jamie his reactions and comments show the meaning he makes of the behavior – a quick abstraction from what Jamie does. Because he sides with Jamie his involvement is different from other staff. The question remains whether or not his interpretation is consistent with the understanding and perspective of the resident.

Not all behavior of the residents can be integrated into patterns. Negative first guesses about a behavior, event, and interaction are essential in the process of coming to understand the residents in their own terms. With inaccurate first guesses and attempts to communicate, the contours of those behaviors which are meaningful can be drawn. Elaborating the boundaries of the individual's pathological behavior provides the opportunity to figure out other ways to describe the individual.

Example 2: Sarah

The description which follows is of an interaction among a teacher, a resident, and the superintendent and gives interpretations from two perspectives. The first interpretation of interaction highlights the difficulty for someone trying to make sense of what is going on. The second interpretation is an alternative version of Sarah's participation from *her* perspective. The example reduces the description of her behavior to her participation in the lesson. This requires an understanding of the nature of what the teacher is doing and the objective for the lesson. Additionally, we need to ask whether the objective corresponds to the nature of Sarah's participation. The superintendent enters the scene with assumptions about what the teacher should be doing.

On this afternoon, after a rest period, the residents going to a puppet show are wheeled down the hall to await the show. A few residents, Patrick, Benjamin, Donald, and Celia return to the activity area; school had been cancelled because of the puppet show and the need for staff assistance to bring the residents to the show. While they are placed on their mats from the wheelchairs by the attendants, a teacher enters with Sarah in a chair. She pushes her over to the mat and takes her out of the chair. Sarah squirms around on the mat, eventually settling herself in the middle, and puts her thumb and index finger into her mouth. She lies quietly. The teacher returns with a full length mirror and props it up against the wall. She leaves again and returns with a comb and a clipboard holding Sarah's program.

The program objective reads: "Sarah will develop the ability to manipulate an object with partial assistance. (a) Demonstrate the ability to keep her head up during the session for a one minute interval. (b) Develop the ability to reach and grasp with partial assistance" (Quarterly educational program report, September 1977).

Since 1977 Sarah has made progress on this objective. She requires partial physical assistance with guidance to manipulate an object rather than total physical assistance.

The teacher retrieves the spoon that Sarah uses to feed herself. She sits down on the mat and places Sarah between her legs. They face the mirror. Sarah bends down over herself. The teacher puts her arms around her, pulls her back up so she faces the mirror directly in full image. The teacher says, "Sarah, pick up the spoon and bring it to your mouth." Sarah faces the mirror but makes no movement. The teacher picks up the spoon and brings it up to her hand. Sarah fingers it but does not grasp. When her fingers are idle, the teacher says, "Bring it to your mouth, like you were going to eat." There was no motion. The teacher sighs. "O.K., here, take the toothbrush." She pulls a toothbrush from a pocket in her blouse and puts it directly into Sarah's hand. As the teacher removes her hand, Sarah lets her own hand fall to the mat. "Pick up the toothbrush," the teacher repeats and waits. Then she wraps her hand around Sarah's hands and together they hold the toothbrush. "Sarah, bring it to your mouth. Brush your teeth." Sarah's head drops. The teacher watches her in the mirror. In a few seconds she lifts her head again.

Sarah is the frequent subject of *petit mal* seizures which last a few seconds to a minute in duration. The frequency of her seizures often interferes with the conduct of her program. "Brush your teeth. Come on, brush your teeth." The teacher guides her own hand and Sarah's hand to Sarah's mouth. When the toothbrush is in her mouth, the teacher exclaims. "Good! That is good." Their hands move up and down together. Behind the teacher, the superintendent of the institution enters the ward. He is on a tour of the building in preparation for an upcoming inspection. As the inspector might do, he bends down to the teacher from behind her and asks, "Excuse me. How are you? Can I ask you what you're doing?" The teacher, astonished at the interruption, looks up at him. Their faces meet eye to eye.

"Yes," she says, acknowledging his greeting but not the question.

"Are you conducting a school program?" The teacher answers, "Yes."

"I see you have the mirror so the resident can see himself." The teacher furrows her brow. He says, "I see you are teaching him to brush his teeth. The mirror is so that he can see himself." The teacher shakes her head.

"No, she can't see, the mirror is there for me. Sarah is blind. The mirror is there so I can see what she is doing."

"Oh," says the superintendent. "She's blind." He walks away. The teacher is bemused and shakes her head. She raises Sarah's hand to her mouth again to brush her teeth. This lasts a few minutes. Then she substitutes a hairbrush on the mat for the toothbrush in Sarah's hand. Bringing it up to her hair, she says, "Now, we are going to brush your hair." When the brush meets the scalp, the teacher takes the hairbrush out of Sarah's hand to brush her hair.

The superintendent walks into the office and starts to check the folders on the residents.

The teacher brushes Sarah's hair for five minutes then picks up the items on the mat, and piles them on the clipboard. She lifts Sarah back into the chair, saying, "Come on, let's get you a treat." She wheels her into the classroom and leaves her for fifteen minutes before delivering some candy M&Ms. It is the evening meal. The teacher wheels her back into the dining area of the activity room, her face smeared from the M&Ms candy with streaks of red, yellow, green, and orange running from the sides of her mouth.

This short sequence illustrates the myriad problems and complications of interpreting what the resident does in an activity. Essentially, the resident is never addressed. The superintendent addresses the teacher and interprets what *she* is doing, not what the resident is doing. He renders an interpretation based on clues in the immediate situation. He assumes knowledge of the situation and the circumstances under which the lesson is conducted before finding out anything about the individual. His assumptions are incorrect; the resident is blind and the mirror is to aid the teacher; the resident is female, not male. Even with difficulties in identification, the assumptions are at best an honest mistake and, at worse, a clumsy one. After the teacher corrects his misunderstanding, he is neither embarrassed nor surprised; he checks that the teacher can answer, not whether he is accurate. The superintendent does not stay to see the activity he has interrupted. His mission is to find out what the residents are doing. He does not go beyond seeing that they *are* enrolled in a school activity and that the activity *is* being conducted.

It is difficult to draw links between statements in educational objectives and the activity as it unfolds, especially in terms of the degree of resident initiative and participation during the lesson. The objective is general and distinguishes assistance in terms of *what the teacher does*, not what the resident should be doing. The reasons for switching from spoon to toothbrush are not clear. Given the general and unspecific nature of the lesson, the substitution of objects and nature of Sarah's handicap, do the events make sense for Sarah?

The teacher has a plan for the lesson to meet the objective. Her substitution of the hairbrush for the toothbrush as an object to grasp is a natural and insignificant change at first glance. But the change represents direction and control within the lesson, exercised by the teacher. Does the substitution have anything to do with Sarah's reaction to the objects? What does her lack of response mean? Performance is assessed in relation to criteria required by the objective, not from the perspective of Sarah's unique skills. Objectives may bring greater specificity to the programs, but gaps will exist if the objectives are not developed from an understanding of the context we create for the teaching of skills.

The series of activities all have elements which fit general parameters of the objective, but it is difficult to draw direct links between the statements in the objective and the activity as it transpires, especially considering the degree of resident initiative and participation during the lesson. When the teacher records comments on the activity, the reasons for the switch from spoon to toothbrush to brush are lost. She records that the resident required total assistance to grasp an object and partial physical assistance to hold up her head.

Within the schema for evaluation of the resident on the objective there is no clear statement of what she can and cannot do. Performance is judged in relation to the criteria of assistance required; what the teacher does, not what the resident feels, experiences or touches. Sarah does not do anything in the activity. Even when the teacher repeatedly exclaims, "Good," there is no evidence in the interaction and Sarah's participation that the resident knows what is happening. "Good" is independent of her participation, as is the switch from spoon to toothbrush to comb. The activity changes at the discretion of the teacher with the introduction of new tasks and objects. With the direction, "Pick up the spoon and bring it to your mouth," the teacher switches spoon for toothbrush. "O.K., here, take the toothbrush," and "Pick up the toothbrush." That the teacher conducts the activity to introduce the objects and the motions to the resident is the most neutral statement of the resident's participation. Evaluation of the activity, then, is best represented in terms of what the resident experiences in the activity rather than in terms of the degree of involvement or assistance provided.

Finally, the teacher gives Sarah a reward, but not in the context of success in the lesson. We do not know if the M&M candy rewards anything in the lesson, but we do learn that when she is left to eat them she is able to grab the candy and bring them to her mouth on her own. Although she has not lifted her hands in the lesson, it is not because she is unable to lift her hand.

Sarah reacts neither to the teacher nor the superintendent nor the spoon nor the toothbrush nor the hairbrushing. She sits motionless. The question arises, what does all this mean for the resident? The mere description of the event leads only to further questions about its meaning. In looking at the resident to understand the event from Sarah's perspective, the description reads differently.

Someone wheels me to another room. I hear Patrick banging his head on the screen. Russel rolls his toy and makes it jingle. Someone pulls me out of my chair and puts me on the mat. I wiggle to get the feel of it. I suck my fingers. I am pulled to someone. Her breast and hair envelop me. Fuzzy long, kinky, hair scratches up against my face as I am bent to my legs by her pushing. I relax and my head falls into my lap. Hearing her talk, I am told something. I startle and open my eyes. I feel something rubber in my hand. I move my fingers around it. I hear someone say something again, I am told something. I feel something plastic in my hand with another hand around mine. When the hand moves away, mine falls to the mat. Someone says something again.

Nothing. My head falls to my chest. I awake. Someone says something. My hand and arm is lifted. My arm swings up. Sharp bristles touch my lips, my teeth and tongue. My hand moves up and down. The voice says something. It continues. The bristles hit my gums. I hear another voice. The two sounds change positions. The hair at my back whisks back and forth across my cheeks, first up and down and then back and forth.

My hand lifts to my mouth and up and down again. My hand moves back to the mat. I feel a smooth handle of plastic. The bristles hit my scalp. I hear the voice. The brush moves around through my hair. Up and down. Up and down. Up and across. Suddenly with a jerk behind me, I fall forward and down onto my legs.

Two hands jab into my armpits. I hear the voice again and feel the arms of my wheelchair and the plastic seat. I move away to a quiet room. I hear something fall on my tray. I swish my hand around and scatter little pebbles. I slap at them. The voice speaks. The round pellets are in my hand. I close my hand and feel the kinky hair. My hand moves to my mouth. The pebbles are on my tongue and in the pockets of my cheeks. The voice speaks again. I slap my teeth together. It is sweet. My tongue swishes to find another pebble. I fish with my hand on the tray. I find some pellets in the corner and surround them with my hand. I close my hand around them and bring them to my mouth. I hit my mouth and open my hand. My tongue hits the hand. Two pebbles smash between my hand and tongue. My hand opens. The taste is everywhere. I lick my hand, wiping it across my face. My tongue moves around, gathering the taste. My hand falls to the tray. Three voices hum in the distance.

Someone rolls me to another space. The wheelchair stops with a jerk. I feel the hair again. I hear voices. Another chair hits my chair. I shake. I sit wiping the tray with my hands.

Two universal social and cultural dimensions to the interactional competence of the severely and profoundly mentally retarded and multiply handicapped may serve as keys to the relationship of the handicap to the person, and as a means to interpret the message of the individual's behavior in context. The first dimension is temporal. Simply, interaction and participation proceed at a different pace. Sarah's pace of interaction is different from that of the teacher. We are not given an indication of Sarah's ability because we are not allowed the opportunity to see her respond. The timing of the lesson is the teacher's and is imposed on Sarah. We do not see what Sarah does because there is no opportunity for her.

The second dimension is spatial. The residents' ability to do – that is, to explore and navigate, to participate in the lesson – is greater than any description of their abilities found within the archive records in the institution or case histories. In this lesson Sarah is encompassed by the hug of the teacher, presumably so that the teacher is able to see what Sarah is doing. This confinement restricts the range for performance by the resident. There is little space for Sarah to respond in the context of the lesson. The residents can only move beyond the boundaries imposed by their handicaps, the institutional rules, adaptive equipment, and the structure of the lesson if there is space to do so. In a physical sense here, restriction of space is symbolic of the need to allow Sarah the opportunity to create her own space, and to explore a range of responses not possible within the teacher's arms.

For example, seeing Sarah's involvement through a revised spatial and temporal framework can help us to see events from her perspective. Such an explanation can enable us to see that Sarah reacts neither to the teacher nor the superintendent nor the spoon, nor to the toothbrush or hairbrush.

She sits motionless. From her perspective, Sarah's non-participation may be understood as a choice not to become involved in the lesson. Teaching skills of independence occurs in a context that fosters dependence. The teacher acts for Sarah and Sarah "cooperates." The message is "I will act for you" or "I will do to you." The teacher's directions to hold another object and exclamation of "good" do not change the nature of her participation but may, in fact, reinforce Sarah's listlessness.

The event is confusing and inconsistent in terms of what Sarah may learn. Basic knowledge of what the severely and profoundly mentally retarded and multiply handicapped do can only be gained from a systematic study of what the residents actually do. Like that of the superintendent and the teacher, our participation is based on assumptions that we know about who they are and what they do. It is not all learned through programs developed by teachers and therapists. The programs are based on our assessment, observation, and understanding of performance. If there are limitations to our understandings, subsequent programs and objectives may be skewed.

Understanding of social context and interactional competence is not a characteristic of the multiple nature of their handicaps but just the opposite. Their patterns of interaction and communication are forged primarily out of living with the handicap and interacting with each other. The patterns in the person's behavior and the handicap exist in relationship to one another. The evolutionary quality of participation of the residents with one another points to the need for a reconciliation of the lesson, methods of observation and assessment, and interpretation of their unique patterns with what the residents do.

Switching from a focus on the handicap to a focus on the individual means that we must relinquish assumptions and expectations that set the individual primarily within the intricacies of the handicap. We must acknowledge a new set of assumptions and expectations: (1) by understanding social context, we can come to understand what individuals do and to appreciate this dimension of their ability; (2) the spatial and temporal dimensions to their behavior require our commitment to understanding the evolutionary nature of their interactions and communicative ability; (3) despite the complicated nature of their handicaps, a message exists in their behavior.

The responsibility for progress is not Sarah's but ours. Sarah should not be asked to figure out the lesson; rather we should be actively engaged in translating and guiding her through the process of exploration and participation in it. It is for us to be surprised by Sarah's ability, not for Sarah to be surprised by our lesson.

Models for understanding

To identify specific communicative purpose, behaviors of the severely and profoundly mentally retarded must be distinguished. Some are redundant; some are whimsical and random; others are initiated to create interest or communicate. Pathological behavior does not communicate. It is a random assortment of mutually inconsistent, sporadic, simultaneously debilitating behaviors. Some behaviors appear over and over again to communicate need. Such behaviors may communicate the necessity to avoid danger, or urgent reactions of fear or pain. Behavior is *social* when any action, behavior, or sequence engages others. The context of interaction determines its social meaning. Knowing the context, we are able to differentiate the following characteristics to the contours of the individual: (1) the ways in which the individual is understandable – the ways in which his or her actions are familiar, recognizable, and identifiable by their demonstration of the shared, learned patterns common to the development of social relationships; (2) the characteristics and the features of the pathology – the ways in which the pathological interferes with and disturbs the formation of social interaction in patterns which can be learned and understood; (3) the overlap between pathological and normal, evident as gradations of pathology and degrees of ability.

Figure 3 illustrates conventional understanding of the difference between the handicapped and the normal. The ways of thinking about difference are shown as two overlapping circles. The circles show the relationship that exists in a human system between the characteristics and features which are normal and those which are pathological.

The circles represent a way of thinking about the handicapped and are intended to force a reconceptualization of the relationship between the individual and the handicap, or the functional ability of the handicapped person. The first circle represents the pathological: those conditions and characteristics which are different and observable and remarkable enough to reveal a fundamental problem in functional ability.

The second circle represents the normal, those "mainstream" ways of looking, acting, behaving, and communicating which are familiar and similar. These are the behaviors and patterns recognizable to staff and parent. Normal is the absence of definable handicapping conditions. Normal is a way of thinking about the ways we act and behave and encompasses biological, human, social, cultural, spiritual, and psychological dimensions. While subtleties and nuances exist in all behavior, the circle represents collective social norms which define the common, acceptable, and understandable and by which the range of variation and differences within a culture and society are determined.

The third area represents the difference, the overlap between the two

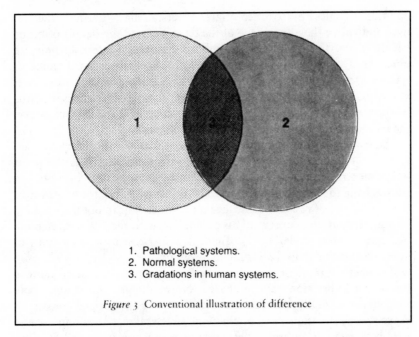

1. Pathological systems.
2. Normal systems.
3. Gradations in human systems.

Figure 3 Conventional illustration of difference

circles. The shaded area is not often defined in terms of the functional ability, but in terms of the handicap. In other words, an individual handicap affects a particular aspect of the human system. Being blind handicaps the individual visually, but need not impair other qualities and characteristics of the individual, nor his or her participation.

In proposing an alternative conceptualization of the relationships between the normal and the pathological, it is necessary to rethink the linear acquisition of skills and behavior management of the individual. The circles illustrate relations between components of the same human system. The severely and profoundly mentally retarded and multiply handicapped communicate understanding in their performance.

Thus the severely and profoundly mentally retarded and the multiply handicapped are individuals whose expression cuts across all three areas in the figure. Some behaviors are pathological: (1) those which are long-term and which incapacitate a particular area of functioning (such as paralysis), (2) those which are short-term and which interfere with performance, (such as a seizure). Understanding the severely and profoundly mentally retarded and the multiply handicapped is a process of differentiating and clarifying the relationship of the handicap to the individual in the context of his or her performance. It requires consideration not only of the characteristics of the handicap, but also of the relative interference of the handicapping condition on performance. The question becomes how to differentiate the person, the actor, the individual over and above the appearance of the disability and the details of his or her daily life. The pathological condition becomes a reference point as much as a departure for understanding performance. As a point of reference, the handicapping condition defines certain limitations to their ability to do things for themselves; but in another sense it defines the basis for further understanding. Performance in context is the key to unravel the relationship between normal and pathological.

The realization that the individual is more than the disability emerges against the background of the handicapping condition. It is the point where the strange becomes familiar: where the guessing born of confusion subsides and the familiar and understandable emerge. It is the point where the foreground of resident behaviors is not the handicap but the meaning of a message in the context of an interaction with the resident. A blink becomes a wink (Ryle, 1971). There is a message in a wink born of acknowledged or shared meaning in a context.

It is when the resident participates in the interaction that the meaning in his or her expression can be shared. Normality for the severely and profoundly mentally retarded and the multiply handicapped consists of those events, situations, and interactions which take on meaning because they have been encountered before: they are recognizable and familiar. They are the ways in which the residents become understandable, not because the exact message is clear, but because the event is recognizable, as when Jamie wheels to sit and thumb through a magazine. This example of what Jamie does invites comparison with other events in which Jamie interacts to arrive at other meanings and interpretations of her ability. The explanation of behavior develops from a hypothesized version in any given situation to an accurate interpretation – by discerning meaning in the patterns of resident behavior which fits the situation.

Behaviors and events and actions are normal for the residents when they are representative and consistent with the actions and behaviors in similar contexts. Normal is what is recognizable and familiar in the conduct of human interaction but also understandable in their own terms – what is normal for them and what they do on their own – whether or not it matches our definition or ideas about what they should be doing. Because of the diversity and complexity of the non-verbal behavior, the characteristics and dimensions of their interactions may not be readily understood.

We can arrive at a meaning for an event by a comparison of different kinds of behavior; that is, we can distinguish the pathological characteristics from attempts to communicate or participate. This categorization process leads to a recognition of patterns in their behavior, which enables us to differentiate meaning. This leads in turn to the identification and

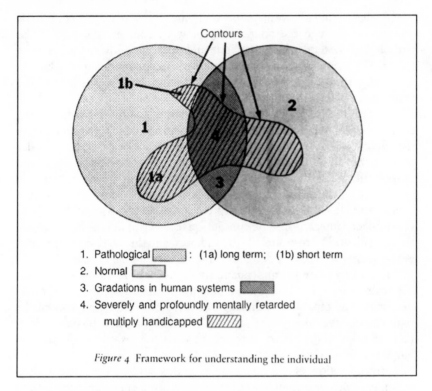

1. Pathological [   ] : (1a) long term; (1b) short term
2. Normal [   ]
3. Gradations in human systems [   ]
4. Severely and profoundly mentally retarded
   multiply handicapped [////]

Figure 4 Framework for understanding the individual

definition of their needs, wants, and desires in their own terms, beyond our assumptions, expectations, and impressions or guesses.

On the overlapping circles of fig. 3 I have superimposed a dynamic model for understanding the severely and profoundly mentally retarded and multiply handicapped as individuals who are not totally pathological, but who exhibit characteristics, expressions, and behaviors which cut into all three areas of the circles (fig. 4). For each individual, a different model can be drawn to represent the unique constellation of characteristics and features. The configuration of the model represents a dynamic relationship between the competing forces of the pathology on one hand and individual expression and behavior on the other.

The contours in fig. 4 represent the dynamic relationship of the handicap to performance. The right circle (2) still represents the normal and familiar. The intersection of circles (1) and (2) in area (3) represents gradations of the handicap and performance ability. The contour that is drawn to represent the individual integrates the whole. The contours represent pathological constraints, both long-term (for example paralysis) and short-term (for example the interruptions of a seizure), but do not isolate these from the other aspects of the individual. The contour is understood through the relationship between competing systems. The pathological systems which debilitate and interrupt performance are one factor. The human system – expressions which communicate and behaviors with purpose – is another factor. In the residents' performance, the systems compete with one another.

The contours are drawn from an understanding of the individual in the context of real life events. For example, consider Jamie's performance in the context of her travels through the apartment. The contours consider performance in all modalities and behaviors which are meaningful and purposeful. What the resident is doing does not fit into a categorical system of classification of behavior. The analysis moves beyond the concrete and linear steps to an interpretation of the behavior in the flow of the resident's interaction. The contours give shape to the configuration of the individual. The contours, the boundaries, and the overlap in the circles evolve from the behavior patterns demonstrated by the individual.

The starting place for understanding the contour is the context of the behavior observed. Through context, the human systems come to be understood as capable of eclipsing one another – the dominance of the pathological over the normal or vice versa. Description of behavior in context helps to determine the effect of what the resident is doing. The handicap influences the execution of behavior.

A consideration of context implies understanding behavior and its meaning as demonstrated by the residents. It is the event, the situation, or the circumstances in which the individual acts which allow differentiation of the pathological behaviors from those which are familiar and are the human dimensions of the individual. Context clarifies the relative influence of the handicap on the individual. How the individual acts in a context defines how the handicap interferes, impedes, obstructs, and challenges the individual in the accomplishment of a task or achievement of a goal.

What is significant is the relationship between purposeful or intentional acts and the restrictions imposed on these acts by the handicap. Also significant is the adaptation the individual makes to the handicap, rather than the handicap itself. Consideration of context provides a different viewpoint from the clinical one in which human experience for the resident is defined for them. Context is where we learn about the individual and what the individual can do. The study of behavior in context can clarify how individuals respond to a situation and how they actively create their social environment.

This model provides a framework for understanding the relationship of the handicap to the person and the relative and dynamic nature by which it influences functional ability. This reconceptualization focuses attention on an individual's functional ability, over and above attributes of the condition identified so clearly by the clinical model. To place responsibility for the limitations of our understanding on our knowledge of their ability, rather than on their pathology, is to make a significant switch in perspective.

3

Residents on their own

The historical context

There is neutral ground on either side of the dividing line, and a person may sometimes be upon the one and sometimes be upon the other, according to the standard of comparison by which he is tried. (Commonwealth of Massachusetts, 1850, 38:34)

Present day categorization of the severely and profoundly mentally retarded and multiply handicapped has historical precedents. Current practice, while trying to align the relationship of the handicapped to the mainstream of society, has not altered the focus of clinical interpretation of pathology which has evolved since the nineteenth century. Traditional interpretations that distinguish normal from abnormal are evident today in other dichotomies: what the individual can and cannot do, or the presence or absence of a particular skill. These are defined without an adequate consideration of context.

From the time of Itard, the feebleminded were studied from a medical clinical perspective. The evolution in the definition of the feebleminded in medicine, psychology, education, and physical anthropology reflects changes over time in the "clinical picture" of the feebleminded.

One important document, a clinical picture of the severely and profoundly mentally retarded and multiply handicapped, is found in the description of custodial cases in Howe's field study (1847), which sought to examine the feebleminded from observation and description of their condition in real life contexts. This firsthand account of the condition of idiots was the forerunner of scientific inquiry into the nature and extent of the problem of feeblemindedness in the United States. Howe sent his fieldworker into the town and communities of the state to investigate, describe, and report on the condition of the feebleminded.

Enos Steven, Howe's fieldworker, rated the characteristics he observed in the feebleminded on a relative mental and physical scale. He observed from half an hour to one hour a day. When information was lacking, secondary sources (relatives and friends) were questioned regarding cause and condition. For the most part, causes were concrete, obvious, and tied to events and circumstances and personal habits. The descriptive data were organized into categories, which in large part classified the material into demographic facts such as age, height, measurements of anatomy, various faculties and specific abilities, and provided a summary of various facts about the family. All the information was gathered to support the *fact* of idiocy, degeneracy, and peculiarities of the feebleminded. These facts, measurements, and relative numerical ratings (0 to 20) of faculties, abilities, and conditions were compiled to support a *case*. Isolated characteristics became attributes of a general classification. Cases were compared for similarity of characteristics of the clinical condition. Later, individuals were referred to by number, and specific cases were cited as examples of Howe's degrees of idiocy. The reduction of fieldnotes to demographic categories constituted the knowledge of that person.

Complex phenomena were reduced by matching characteristics with labels. Categories chopped relationships into entities related in content but isolated by the boundaries of the definition. Because of the general survey nature of the fieldnotes, there were problems in interpreting any individual's functional ability.

The harmonious relations between the person and the soul, which Howe so strongly championed, were lost in facts, attributes, categories, and measurements. Behaviors, facilities and abilities were classified as single entities divorced from their conditions and contexts. A numerical rating provided only a *relative* standard for interpretation of the categories as one pieced together what the person actually could do. Consider the description of Case 410, synthesized by Howe from the fieldnotes. The case exemplifies the fact of idiocy but not what the person could do.

No. 410. E. G. aged 8 years. This poor creature may be taken as a type of the lowest kind of idiocy. He has bones, flesh and muscles, body and limbs, skin, hair, etc. He is, in form and outline, like a human being, but in nothing else. Understanding he has none; and his only *sense* is that which leads him to contract the muscles of his throat, and swallow food when it is put into his mouth. He cannot chew his victuals; he cannot stand erect; he cannot even roll over when laid upon a rug; he cannot direct his hands enough to brush off the flies from his face; he has no language – none whatever; he cannot even make known his hunger, except by uneasy motions of his body. His habits of body are those of an infant just born. He makes a noise like that of a very sick and feeble baby, not crying however in a natural way. His head is not flattened and deformed, as is usual with idiots, but it is of good size and proportion.

It would seem as if the powers of *innervation* were totally wanting in him. There is no more power of *contractility* than in a person who is dead drunk. The involuntary muscular motions are properly performed; that is, the organic life goes on regularly; the heart contracts and dilates; the peristaltic motion of the bowels is regular.

The probable causes are hereditary ones. The grandparents were very scrofu-

lous and unhealthy. The parents were apparently healthy, but gave themselves up
to excessive sensual indulgence. They lost their health in consequence of this, and
were so well aware of it as to abstain and to recover again. In the meantime, five
children were born to them – two of whom were like E. G., and died at five or six
years of age: two others were very feeble and puny and died young. (Commonwealth of Massachusetts, 1848:61–62)

Howe stated, "The born idiot remains an idiot" (Howe, 1870:6)
Warning against misuse of the general definition, Howe thought
feeblemindedness encompassed the following characteristics:

Without pretending, then, to any scientific accuracy, idiocy may be defined to be
that condition of a human being in which, from some morbid cause in the bodily
organization, the faculties and sentiments remain dormant or undeveloped, so
that the person is incapable of self-guidance, and of approaching that degree of
knowledge usual with others of his age. (Commonwealth of Massachusetts,
1848:20)

Howe believed that the obvious functions of the brain were determined
by physical attributes. In other words, the limited size of the brain was
indicative of an equally small capacity for self-governance. A concrete
relationship existed between anatomical features and functional
capacity. Diminished capacity made the need for schooling and provisions for lifelong care obvious. Convinced of society's obligation, he
was steadfastly committed to the cultivation of the individual by
training.

Howe was aware of the dangers of a classification scheme developing as
a caste. "Nature produces individual men, not classes" (Commonwealth
of Massachusetts, 1850, 38:33). Nevertheless, he proposed subclasses of
the feebleminded to describe distinct groups within the definition based on
observable functional differences. Howe maintained a curious sensitivity
to the action, reaction and interaction of various functions of the brain.
Discriminating functional abilities, he sought to determine a classification
scheme for the various degrees of idiocy. The features of idiocy for Howe
were: (1) the organic nature of the disease and its manifestations, (2)
functional ability, and (3) the effect of each on the intellectual and moral
character of the individual. The potential for the harmonious mix of all
three for the individual was limited, but the *imperfect combination of all*
three was limitless.

For example, Howe distinguished idiots from fools. Idiot was the
lowest functioning classification at the time of the study. In short, idiots
were "without any manifestation of intellectual or affective faculties,"
and "Fools are a higher class of idiots ... who have partial development of
the affective intellectual faculties, but only the faintest glimmer of reason,
and very imperfect reason." (Commonwealth of Massachusetts,

1848:61). The faintest glimmer of reason, intellect and affect he considered to be demonstrated in "another kind of language" (p. 68). This remarkable insight was an early reference to the fact that the feebleminded themselves may possess another kind of "propensity for expression."

Howe drew attention to the lack of moral character as a feature of idiocy. The combination of unharmonious faculties impeded the development of moral character. This added an implication to the description of idiocy which was consistent with socially held beliefs and the popular conception at the time: namely, that the feebleminded were the cause of degeneracy and criminal activity.

Howe believed that idiocy was the result of and a punishment for parental sin. Idiocy was a consequence of the violation of the "natural" laws of humanity and those violations included intemperance, moral impropriety, close intermarriage among family members, and the transmission of hereditary disease. Of the 574 individuals he studied, 420 were classified as congenital idiots, and from information gathered in interviews gained from family members, the condition of 359 of the total was said to be due to some violation or sin.

Will was an independent factor that operated within the biological and intellectual constraints of idiocy. Howe argued for the skillful guidance of the individual and management of the handicap so as not to frustrate the will of the individual.

Howe warned that intense scrutiny of individual attributes did not constitute a description of the fundamental uniqueness of each individual personality – the *soul*. Measurement and inspection did not constitute nor capture this unique characteristic.

It is a matter of great importance that those to whom the care of feebleminded children is entrusted, should understand thoroughly the distinction between *organic* and *functional* defects in the brain ... The *treatment* of the brain is, however, a very difficult and delicate task. We sometimes want to bring one of its organs into action, and at the same time to repress undue activity in another. Great tact and discrimination are here required, lest we confound one organ with another, and thus do more harm than good ... It is also very important that the brain, its organs, and its functions should not be confounded with the soul, its faculties and its attributes ... A man has a brain and a set of cerebral organs. If these organs are found to exist in due number and proportion, and are all in good order, the combined action resulting from their character will be harmonious. If they are not, then it will not. Now, the brain and its organs do not constitute the soul ... The soul – the incomprehensible man – sits behind the brain, and plays upon it, as the musician plays upon the instrument. People of uncultivated minds are apt to mistake a function of the brain for a faculty of the soul, and an error of the kind may render all efforts to train and educate an idiotic person futile and unsuccessful. (Howe 1875: 21–23)

Scattered throughout Howe's supplemental report (Commonwealth of Massachusetts, 1848) was mention of the fact that the fools he was observing demonstrated natural signs. Howe explains his concept of these "natural signs":

the external sign by which such internal structure and condition can be known, is as much the natural language of passion as a smile is the natural language of gladness. Now, to say that, because such signs have not yet been satisfactorily ascertained, therefore they never can be ascertained, and that the attempt to ascertain is impious or foolish, is just what it would have been a few years ago to say that, because a nebula never had been resolved, therefore it never could be resolved; that infusoria never had been seen, and therefore, never could be seen; and that to turn a telescope to the sky, or the microscope to the water, was impious and foolish. (Commonwealth of Massachusetts, 1848:68)

In fieldnotes on Case 35 (Jonas), Stevens noted:

The whole lateral region of the brain on both sides is at a high fever heat and he is most impetuous and furious and exercises, at full liberty, the most voracious and vitiated appetite for all sorts of food. He will even swallow chips, bark, raw potatoes, carrots [?] out of the swill pail, though he has eaten what he chooses at a well furnished table. He often swallows pebbles as large as common chestnuts. (Howe, 1847)

Stevens concluded "he has a very idiotic appearance about the eyes and the mouth," and, significantly, he added: "He does not use words, but has considerable signs of ideas and understands much that is said to him."

Another example in which natural signs are described is Case 360.

No. 360, George, Pauper. He seems to have little or no command over the motions of the body. He is very paralytic, and at the same time continually distorted by various involuntary spasms, which move him slowly and seem to crawl along his limbs. He was puny from birth; early practiced masturbation, was gluttonous, had fits and spasms, and never could walk or do anything of any consequence except hold a spoon or fork to feed himself. All his joints are most terribly drawn out of shape, and seem to be all bent back the wrong way, his parents were most drunken, scrofulous, and little able or willing to provide for him. Yet he seems to know much that is going on around him, talks some so as to be understood, but slowly. He has very extraordinary powers of reckoning, so that he can tell how many seconds old any one is, in a few minutes. (Howe, 1847)

The fieldnotes, the numerical ratings, and the report (Commonwealth of Massachusetts 1848) which Howe provided did not address the possibilities of integration between these characteristics of the organic and functional, the will and soul. His categories did not allow a description of performance and expression hinted at in the fieldnotes. Clinical, categorical selectivity, not only by the observer but also in the categories themselves, was problematic. In a strange and fascinating twist of logic, the very means by which he hoped to describe the individual – categories of characteristics – failed to account for the very basic and most fundamental expression of the self. A comparison of relations and links between the categories produces, in the case of the Howe study, sets of categorical facts about the feebleminded.

Characteristics relative to ability and the degree and type of idiocy do not negate the will of the individual. The individual's forms of expression, the natural signs representing the soul of the individual are significant features by which to identify who the individual is and what he does. For Howe, education and intervention had to be provided in such a way as to fulfil the will of the individual.

Subsequent inquiry into the life of the mentally retarded was to be grounded, not in the natural expressions and signs, but rather in the model of the case study exemplified by Itard and the clinical approach to education advocated by Séguin. Maria Montessori (1870–1952) acclaimed Itard's work as the original application of experimental psychology. Montessori believed that the future development of the feebleminded was not only through surgery or medical intervention but also through education and training. She attempted to apply the medical clinical model to the design of instruction. The feebleminded were chiefly a pedagogical problem (Montessori, 1912:13).

Montessori developed one of Séguin's themes in her advocacy of a total picture of the individual through the case study:

Taking measurements of the head, the stature, etc. (in other words, applying the anthropological method), is, to be sure, not in itself the practice of pedagogy but it does mean that we are following the path that leads to pedagogy, because we cannot educate anyone until we know him thoroughly. (Montessori, 1913:17)

If the medical, psychological and anthropological study of congenital abnormalities established a biological basis of variation from the norm, then pathological anthropology became the study of ontogenic development of man and the range of variation within the characteristics considered normal. Anthropology assisted medicine with the inspection and measurement of physical attributes. The accumulation of computations of the biological features from abnormal and normal individuals provided a comparative standard. To observe and measure objectively, Montessori stated that the observer must divest himself of the preconceptions of normal and abnormal. The anthropologist must perform the anthropometry without knowing if the child was educated or illiterate (Montessori, 1913:24–25). The teacher provided additional observations. Through cooperation with the teacher and the physician, the anthropologist helped to advance the perfection of man and the entire culture by evolving practical rules for the practice of education.

The ambitious goal Montessori set for pedagogic anthropology was the moral and hygienic education of students. A rational method of diagnosis and clinical judgement was to support the selection and segregation of deviant populations (feebleminded and delinquent) – a first step towards the perfection of mankind. The aim was to increase the understanding of the normal through the study of deviant features. Despite the benevolence of these goals, this careful diagnosis meant separation and segregation for some based on the measurement of physical characteristics.

At this point in history, the contribution that anthropology made to medicine and education was the understanding of the human species, awareness of human evolution and variation to clarify standards of normality. Gradually, a shift in thinking occurred, which tried to understand the "normal" in human nature rather than the variation. The understanding of the normal attributes of the human species became the best means of understanding the differences. This shift used biological norms and characteristics to classify those who were different. Once the norms were established, they were used to classify. Anthropometry itself became the tool in the measurement and the classification of the feebleminded.

The scientific study of the feebleminded continued over the turn of the century, as institutions for their care and treatment proliferated and society grew more concerned about the general causes and conditions of degeneracy. Laboratories were set up within the institutions to examine every facet of feeblemindedness. The anthropometric examination and laboratory were founded, based on the optimistic premise that the measurement and the determination of relations between organs would lend itself to accurate diagnosis and early identification.

Although anthropological examination of the feebleminded was initiated with grand hopes of understanding human variation, all it managed to do was to complement medical practice with descriptions of the feebleminded (Doll, 1916; Fernald *et al.*, 1918). The measurement of physical features to determine specific characteristics and attributes, an innovation at the turn of the century, resulted in the collection of specimens and skeletons, autopsy reports and body measurements. In the research units and laboratories emerging within the institutions, attention turned to psychological, metabolic and genetic causes of feeblemindedness.

The directions taken by research to understand the causes of feeblemindedness went beyond the physical and the biological. Pedigree studies were initiated to show that idiocy was inherited. Pictures of clinical characteristics were used to identify criminals and exclude immigrants. The investigator sought explanations in external factors and variables, for example the effect of birth order and astrology. The explanation of feeblemindedness became in the public mind the degeneracy, crime and prostitution of the parents.

The establishment of intelligence as a single, statistically measured entity provided the numerical basis for degrees and types of feeblemindedness.

The study of general intelligence and the characteristics of mental ability was introduced by Alfred Binet (1857–1911). Binet, expanding the biological medical model into a "psychological model," assembled a group of tasks to analyze and measure the structures and faculties of human thinking.

The principle of classification of the feebleminded by degree or type of idiocy was forever changed with the advent of the intelligence test score. Within the classification system, which up to this time had been descriptive, the degree of idiocy became associated with a fixed intelligence test score, in which numerical values distinguished one level of feeblemindedness from another.

Lewis Terman (1879–1956) popularized intelligence testing in America, basing his campaign on certain assumptions. He assumed that the general test score was an *entity* – that is, general intelligence – and that intelligence was *innate*. In these statistical formulations, a score represented the relationship between mental age and chronological age, as well as standard deviation from this score. Thus intelligence testing provided a scientific, statistical measure to legitimize the "psychological method" refined by Binet, the mental analogue to the medical and clinical examinations which defined syndromes.

The clinical identification of syndromes was underscored in the establishment of intelligence quotients for particular syndromes. The descriptions of particular cases now included a rich listing of the syndrome's physical characteristics and features, and an assessment of intellectual ability based on performance of particular tasks. The popular mismeasure of the feebleminded ("mismeasure" because of the belief that the test measured a single entity) became the intelligence test, but also established the degree of feeblemindedness (Gould, 1981). Intelligence, or the innate reasoning capacity as measured by tests, became a predictor of ability to participate in school and society.

Measurement of intelligence began in America with testing, not observation. Mental measurement provided a scale numerical value by which to classify types and degrees of feeblemindedness. Measurement complemented the medical model and scientific experimental model. The population of severely and profoundly mentally retarded and multiply handicapped were at the extreme end of the continuum where performance on a test was unthinkable. Such individuals were labelled "untestable" by default, for nonperformance, rather than for the successful administration of the test items.

PROFOUND MENTAL RETARDATION, a term used to describe the degree of retardation present when intelligence test scores are below 20 or 25; such persons require continuing and close supervision, but some persons may be able to perform simple self-help tasks; profoundly retarded persons often have other handicaps and require total life-support systems for maintenance. (Grossman, 1983:184)

Terms such as "mental deficiency," "feeblemindedness," "mental subnormality," and "mental handicap," based on a reevaluation of the functional abilities, were used to describe a population. A universally accepted definition was the result of these reconsiderations of levels and sublevels of mental retardation: "Mental retardation refers to subaverage general intellectual functioning which originates in the developmental period and is associated with impairment in adaptive ability." The emphasis was on "natural and social demands in his environment. Impaired adaptive behavior may be reflected in: (1) maturation, (2) learning and/or (3) social adjustment" (Heber, 1961:3).

This general definition was provided by a combination of the medical classification, the etiological characteristics of the condition, and acknowledgement of behavioral and psychological functions including levels of adaptive behavior, measured intelligence, and personal social development.

The heterogeneous factors studied and included in the 1961 definition made by the American Association of Mental Deficiency – the professional authority within the United States for determining classification – were a categorical maze, through which a path had to be picked to discover the combination of etiological systems, mental categories, intelligence quotients, and adaptive behavior patterns. Increased emphasis on functional and adaptive behavior and severity found its place in the definition of the severely and the profoundly mentally retarded. Performance potential in self-help skills was acknowledged, along with the fact that increased life support might be required. Short life expectancy no longer remained the sole prognosis.

Resident socialization

This definition of mental retardation by means of the dividing line described by Howe in 1850 continued to support the dichotomy of normal and abnormal with increasing specificity, but it did not change the underlying conceptualization. A reconceptualization begins with integration of the clinical definition of the characteristics of the condition with performance within specific contexts. With knowledge of clinical constraints, performance ability is highlighted in what an individual does on his own and with others. To see such individuals' ability within a specific context diminishes the significance of the dividing line. The question is not whether they are normal or abnormal, but rather what individuals do in context, given the constraints of their pathological condition.

The examples of Danial and Thomas which follow focus attention on such a view of ability. To see their ability, we observe the natural signs, expression, and language in their attempt to do something. Interpretation of ability proceeds from the reconceptualization to an identification of patterns in what they do.

The evolution of a pattern depends on the repetition of a behavioral repertoire in similar circumstances. The individual becomes known in the social environment by the activation of a consistent behavioral repertoire – for example the patterns in Thomas's and Danial's play with a lawn mower. Whether the patterns in behavior are shared or social depends on the consistency with which the resident demonstrates the behavior, the cooperation he receives from others, staff or residents, and the choices the resident makes.

The constitutive elements of the social behavior between Danial and Thomas as well as other residents include the following: (1) An inter-action is situation dependent – for example, residents are placed together on a mat fortuitously. (2) The behavior of one resident attracts the attention of the other and invites a response, for example, reaching for a toy. (3) The invitation gets a response. (4) The cycle of invitation–response repeats itself. Whether this cycle is allowed to evolve depends on interruptions by staff enforcing rules of the apartment or structuring a lesson, or complications of the handicapping conditions. More often than not, it is the staff's involvement with the residents which is problematic. (5) The residents' interaction survives interruptions – for example, the play between Thomas and Danial. It evolves into a pattern to achieve a recognizable outcome. This definition can be learned through the con-struction of the interaction. That is, the behavior of the resident evolves into patterns that are shared and learned, are understandable to other residents, and are recognizable to staff.

The residents experience the full breadth of human expression within the constraints of their handicap and the environment in which they live. The context for the interaction or event determines its social meaning. The messages contained within their behavior are the signs of what they are doing and can be understood through the consideration of context. In the following example, the context is the rest period. The event is in one sense what these two residents "get away with."

The descriptions which follow illustrate a range of interactional behav-ior and events in which the residents participated during the conduct of the study. The examples focus on qualities of the interaction between the residents, the richness in their ability to participate in play when left to

themselves, the complexity of their involvement and execution of movements and behaviors, the simple enjoyment inherent in activities and
events when they engage each other. The descriptions also demonstrate
purposeful and intentional qualities in their behavior. These are of course
not the only examples of residents' behavior, nor are they illustrative of
the entire range and the depth of each resident's ability. Not all of the
residents play and socialize in the manner described below. Each resident
demonstrates his own interactional ability and participatory ability
within the constraints of disability on functioning. What each resident
demonstrates is the ability to understand and act in social interactions
with others.

This event occurs in the activity area in apartment M and N during the first
period of observation on the afternoon of a staff party for Saint Patrick's Day.

On this day, the foster grandmothers roll residents up and down the hall,
some with green shamrocks in lapel buttons and blouses. About twenty
residents are still on the ward, each positioned in a sandbag chair or mat, or
triangular wedge. Kenneth rolls his rubber duck in and out of his hand. June
screams after she is changed; an attendant who quiets her yells at her jokingly,
"Crazy June, why don't you shut up!" Some attendants take turns going down
the hall to spend time at the party. Others watch the residents.

Irritated at June's continual slapping of her face and screaming, one attendant
walks down to her at the other end of the hall and holds her hands down. A
second attendant, observing the scene, comments to her, "Stop beating up on
June."

"O.K., when she shuts up."

Two people walk in to look at a wheelchair. The tall young attendant passes
Thomas on the edge of the mat, as he is pushing a Fisher-Price lawn mower out
into the aisles between the mats. She pauses and says to him, "Now Thomas,
don't be pushing that out [into the aisle]." Thomas smiles. She repeats more
emphatically, "Now don't," as he continues to roll it off the mat. She walks by
and on to June. Somehow the lawn mower finds itself in the aisle.

Another older woman attendant finds the toy in the aisle and says to the
red-headed attendant who just returned with her from the party, "They will kill
for this toy." I don't know who she means, but decide to pay attention to the
toy's whereabouts. The two attendants walk around the toy towards the office.
Before arriving, they find Celia in her wheelchair about to bump into the
outstretched hands of Patrick collecting his rubber toys. "Will you get out of
here!" the attendant exclaims as she grabs hold of Celia's wheelchair handles
and turns her away from Patrick. "She's going to run his hands off." She
pushed the chair toward the bedroom door, "Will you get out of here!"

Celia smiles, as she rolls in the opposite direction but stops herself before the
doorway by dragging her right foot on the floor and her hands on the wheel.

This two-and-a-half-hour continuous play event occurred in March 1978.
The toy found in the aisle by the attendants is the object of play for the

entire sequence of events. Thomas's favorite toy was identified by staff in November 1979. By this time, teachers said in passing, "Hello, Thomas, I see that you have your favorite toy." Attendants also make comments about the toy, "That's his lawn mower. We're going to have him doing lawns during the summer time."

Each attendant points out a salient feature of the interaction. The first identifies the fact that toys are not to be kept in the aisle: the residents are told to keep them on the mat. In this interaction the attendants attribute to the residents the ability to understand verbal statements of the rules. Second, the toy they will "kill for" is a Fisher-Price lawn mower. This comment, even in jest, implies behavior which should be stopped, controlled, which is potentially harmful, and misrepresents the nature of their interaction. That the boys and other residents will play with the toy is nothing new. Reference to a favorite toy is found in each boy's records. As one attendant remarks, "Everyone's got one little thing they're supposed to have."

The grandmother who takes Danial on walks after lunch returns him. She asks him if he liked seeing the party and wheels into the first mat by the door. The two attendants lift Danial down onto the mat next to Thomas lying there quietly. Both Thomas and Danial lie on their back (supine position) as their natural and preferred position. (Both accomplish the interactions to be described from the supine position except where described in the text.) The grandmother left the lawn mower in the aisle, but the attendant places it on the mat next to Danial, and in between him and Thomas. Danial does not look over towards Thomas, but soon begins to pull at the string suspended from the line hung across the length of the activity area. A doll hangs from the string. He rubs the body of the doll with one hand, his other hand tucked beneath him. His hand falling from the doll, Danial grabs at the Fisher-Price lawn mower to his right. The toy has a wooden handle, attached to a plastic cylinder with colored balls inside. When rolled across a surface, plastic wheels on either side of the cylinder turn plastic blades inside it. Colored balls fly in all directions. The wheels activate a musical disc that repeats a ditty over and over. When rolled, the lawn mower provides a display of popping colored balls that seem to accompany the tune.

Danial moves his hand up the handle, wraps his hand tightly around it, and lifts the lawn mower up over his head. It almost lands on his forehead because of the weight of the cylinder. He quickly compensates for the sway of the lawn mower towards his head by sliding his hand up the middle of the handle. He halts the lawn mower not more than half-an-inch from his head. Recovering control of the toy, he immediately forces it back up the arc of its fall, aiming toward the suspended doll. He misses the doll. The weight swiftly brings the lawn mower down on the other side onto the mat, out of his hand, brushing the side of his leg.

Danial reaches up and pulls at the doll. The line shakes from the pull. He lets go. The doll bounces around in space above him. As Danial reaches for the handle of the lawn mower, he moves off the mat. By gripping the floor with his left arm curled underneath him and pressing down, he generates friction between himself and the floor, lifts up from his hand, dragging his body behind him. He also uses his right arm to push off. Because it does not curl under him like his left, he can reach further. This time he uses both hands to slide himself off the mat.

Danial slides across the mat into the aisle in pursuit of the lawn mower. He rolls over towards the lawn mower by tucking his right arm underneath him, transferring all his weight to his right side as he turns his head and left shoulder. He uses his feet to push off, extending the sole of the right foot flat against the floor to lift up. He uses his left leg to transfer weight to his right side. With most of the weight shifted to his right side, his body topples over so he lies on his stomach. To recover from the turn, he turns his head to the side, props himself up again on his right side, and looks at the object he rolled toward, the lawn mower.

From the position on his side, Danial lifts the lawn mower over his head like a flag. It falls over his body onto the other side of the mat. He turns back over, reversing the moves he made to follow the lawn mower. He has trouble making a complete turn. With a straining neck and a grunting noise to punctuate the energy expended, he finally makes the move. He flops over and a smile crosses his face. He picks up the lawn mower by the handle, holds it vertically.

Although the attendants comment on the value of the toy, they do not place the toy on the mat or give it to Thomas. Danial's placement on the first mat next to Thomas is a fortuitous placement for both boys. The grandmother sets the Fisher-Price lawn mower between the two boys. All three individuals attending to Danial's move walk away without a word. They place him on the mat and leave.

On the mat, Danial immediately hits a doll suspended above him with the lawn mower. Danial swings at the doll in a consistent and persistent fashion. He demonstrates ability to manipulate a tool. He compensates for the weight of the lawn mower by positioning his hand.

Then two attendants come out of the office and look down at Thomas who has crawled into the middle of the aisle. Without saying a word, they bend down and pick him up, sighing, "Come on." They bring him to another mat across the room, their feet shuffling across the floor, holding him by the arms and underneath the knees. Danial collapses between them. When the attendant says, "O.K., that's enough," they stop at the closest mat and place him down on it. They walk about thirty feet from where he has been to the other end of the activity area and out the rear door to return to the party. Another attendant sits in the office.

Hardly a few seconds have elapsed when Thomas starts to move across the mat onto the floor. Danial is now using the lawn mower as a mallet to hit the doll. He raises the lawn mower in his left hand and swings at the doll. When he misses, the lawn mower falls to the mat or onto his leg. This time he never lets the lawn mower get out of control nor lets it go. Sometimes he nicks the doll, and it spins around. He makes five good tries in the space of ten minutes. Thomas has moved himself off the mat and into the aisle and is still moving, heading back to his original position.

For the next 20 minutes, Thomas moves across the floor slowly, half-inch by half-inch without stopping to rest, each movement in synchrony with the next. In slow, accordion-like movements, pulling together and pushing out his entire body, he propels himself across the tiles of the floor. In his long journey around mats and down aisles, he moves around a sandbag chair in the aisle. Regaining the lost ground, he returns to the point from which he was moved. Thomas pauses as an attendant comes out of the office a distance of six to eight feet away from Danial.

Danial himself has moved off the mats into a position in the aisle that Thomas is coming down. With each roll, he carefully maintains his hold on the lawn mower.

The attendant comes out of the office and sees Danial. She looks at him and says, "They'll do anything for that toy." She passes on to inspect the others. With no word between them, a second attendant comes from the sleeping area, walks past Danial, stops to look at Thomas, who stops moving as soon as the first attendant enters the room. She stoops down to rub his stomach; he looks up from the floor and watches her. Next, she goes to get a second lawn mower on a distant mat, returns and gives it to Thomas. As she gives it to him, she says, "This is their favorite toy. They all like it." Thomas smiles.

Two attendants move Thomas from the aisle out of the way and onto another mat to comply with the rule that residents are to be on the mats at all times. They perform the duty perfunctorily without discussion.

Thomas moves across the floor a distance of thirty feet to resume his position. Thomas inches himself forward in a series of slow deliberate movements. He pauses when an attendant appears at the office door and resumes his travels as she moves out of sight.

Danial moves off the mat into the aisle, positioning himself almost directly in the line of Thomas's movement. The first attendant states she is aware that they will do anything for the toy, even crawl a long distance making difficult moves. A second attendant stoops to rub Thomas's stomach. She brings another toy with her and gives it to him.

Danial and Thomas move toward one another. At first the toy is the focus of their attention. Having the toy is not the sole motivation, however.

In a series of three rolls, Danial finds himself head-to-toe with Thomas. Thomas maneuvers parallel to Danial. Thomas's legs angle behind him. Danial's legs rest just to one side of Thomas's head. Each holds a lawn mower. Each brings it around in front of him to hold parallel to the other. Looking into each other's knees, they can look down the length of the other's torso to see the second lawn mower. The toys and their hands appear to obstruct direct eye contact.

Danial has the white-handled lawn mower and Thomas the blue-handled lawn mower. The toys are identical. Danial lifts the white-handled lawn mower up to and over his face. It shields his face. With this, Thomas grips the blue-handled lawn mower resting loosely in the palm of his hand. He inches closer to and down towards the chest and head of Danial and within an arm's length of Danial's white handled lawn mower. As Thomas is moving down towards him, Danial takes the lawn mower down from his face and pushes it toward Thomas, who grits his teeth. Danial quickly withdraws it. Thomas himself moves in closer to Danial, positioning his lawn mower next to Danial's. Letting his own drop to the floor, Thomas quickly reaches for the white handle of Danial's lawn mower. Danial pulls it back toward him as soon as Thomas lunges toward it. A moment elapses in which neither one does anything except stare. Then Danial pushes the lawn mower towards Thomas while moving himself away from Thomas. Thomas grabs at the white handle but cannot get it out of Danial's grip. Maintaining his grip Danial reaches over and tries to grab the blue handle of Thomas. Danial misses. Neither one has succeeded in grabbing the other's toy. Thomas slowly reaches for the white handle of the lawn mower. Suddenly, he dramatically throws himself towards Danial and grabs the white-handled lawn mower. In the process, he jerks back quickly, pushing his own blue-handled lawn mower away from him. Recovering from the movement, he drags the white-handled lawn mower from Danial. Danial seizes the opportunity to grab the blue handle of Thomas's lawn mower, and pulls it swiftly back towards himself, keeping an eye on Thomas. Then with a smile, he lifts the blue-handled lawn mower over his head, holds it in a flag position, and then lets it drop to the floor. Thomas turns his head away from Danial and rolls the white-handled lawn mower on the floor beside him. The musical ditty plays and Thomas watches the balls jump in the cylinder, ignoring Danial.

A second exchange begins. Again, Danial lifts the blue-handled lawn mower over his head. Ignoring him, Thomas holds the white-handled lawn mower to his side and away from Danial, by two feet. Danial eases the lawn mower to the floor. Turning the wheel and the cylinder towards himself, he uses the handle to poke into the ribs of Thomas. With each poking motion, Thomas moves a little further away, rolls his eyes and grits his teeth. Danial continues to poke at him with a developing smile. Thomas drops the white-handled lawn mower, reaches across his body and grabs at the handle of the lawn mower poking him. The handle slides through his fingers as he fails to close his grip. There is just enough time for Danial to slide the lawn mower away from him. Danial is grinning. Thomas moves the white-handled lawn mower back between them and rolls it. Then with his full arm extended, he picks it up and holds it over Danial's head. Danial, in one swoop, drops the lawn mower he holds and reaches for the lawn mower over his head. He misses it. The arm and lawn mower pass each other unimpeded. Thomas, humming and smiling, withdraws the lawn mower slowly from over Danial's head. In his swing, Danial has pushed the blue-handled lawn mower into the open space between them with his body. He reaches directly and swiftly for the blue handle of the lawn mower and pulls it close beside him, the cylinder next to his chest and the handle underneath his thigh.

Thomas's reciprocal move is to reach out. Putting a hand against Danial's shoulder, he pushes him away with a grunting noise. Thomas follows by moving himself away. They increase the distance between them by two or three feet. Having held on to the white-handled mower on the floor in front of him, Danial watches Thomas holding his own lawn mower close to his chest. Danial rolls the blue-handled lawn mower towards Thomas, pushing slowly and gradually. Initially, Thomas appears unconcerned, then he drops the handle of his lawn mower and grabs the approaching one. He misses and picks up the white-handled toy again and rolls it into Danial's chest. The surge of the movement extends him far beyond his reach and he loses the lawn mower. Danial, who has been hit, drops his own lawn mower.

Both boys move into a position symmetrical to one another and begin a rapid fire exchange of toys. The different colors on each lawn mower's handle flag the reciprocity in the event. Both boys exchange an object after a mutual challenge and attempt to get what the other has; then retrieve what the other boy has taken, a mutual exchange and recovery. Pushing the toy in the direction of the other is a challenge and an invitation.

With the placement of the two toys between them, Thomas moves first to lunge at the white handle of Danial's mower. Danial just as quickly withdraws it. The second exchange begins when Danial, taking the initiative, rolls the lawn mower out towards Thomas. The second exchange is quite dramatic in its speed and in Thomas's resourcefulness. He sneaks up on Danial in a series of barely perceptible movements. Although Thomas successfully takes the lawn mower away from Danial, he loses his own. Danial holds the blue-handled toy over his head as if triumphant, spoiling the victor's pleasure. Thomas takes little notice and turns away from Danial. Seemingly oblivious, Thomas rolls the lawn mower at his side.

At the beginning of the first exchange, raising and lowering the lawn mower like a flag seems to be like an independent gesture on the part of Danial. With the initiation of the second exchange, the use of the toy is more like a signal to play. When this does not work, Danial uses the toy to prod Thomas into action. The goading causes an immediate reaction. Thomas jerks away, gritting his teeth. He dislikes the provocation and reacts. When Thomas reaches out to grab Danial's lawn mower, he demonstrates displeasure and does something about it. Danial's quick reaction in pulling away from Thomas reveals another link between the two. Danial grins, Thomas holds the lawn mower over Danial as a threat or a warning. Danial takes the gesture as a challenge. This time Thomas hums and smiles. Each prompts and challenges the other. Each movement invites a counter-action by the other. The exchange is provocative but mutual.

In the next series of interchanges in the event, each boy tries to sneak up on the other while guarding his own toy. Thomas grabs hold of the approaching lawn mower and pushes it into Danial's chest. Each boy relinquishes his lawn mower in the space between them. Each observes momentary calm.

The two lawn mowers lie side by side in the space on the floor between the two boys. The two are startled by the turn of events. Thomas moves closer to the toys, picks up the white-handled lawn mower and pushes it into Danial's stomach. After the jab, he picks it up and swings it over Danial's head. It wavers and falls close to Danial, but never touches his head. Danial does not reach for the toy over his head, but for the blue-handled toy in front of him. He pushes it toward Thomas. With this, Thomas withdraws the white-handled toy from over Danial's head.

Precisely at the time the toys are being withdrawn, an attendant enters the activity area from the office, looks down at the boys and says, "What are you fighting for?" She at once separates Thomas from Danial. She picks up Thomas by sliding her arms underneath his armpits, bending him up to her waist and dragging him across the floor a distance of twelve feet, with his legs trailing behind him. Danial immediately pulls the blue-handled lawn mower into his chest to protect it and shield it from sight. As he is being lifted, Thomas grabs for his own white-handled lawn mower, just in time to maintain it. The attendant returns and picks up Danial in the same fashion, to move him away from Thomas. Unwittingly, although she tries to distance them from one another, she places them on mats almost directly across from each other and separated only by the aisle.

Each boy drops his toy in the aisle between the mats, unable to sustain a grip. Thomas drops his while hunched over and bent from the attendant's position. It lands in the aisle. The attendant pushes Danial's lawn mower out of his hand when it wedges between them on the move. Danial lets go just on the edge of the mat.

On the mat, Danial immediately rolls over in the direction opposite to the toys and toward the wall into the sunshine. Thomas, on the other hand, moves into the aisle between the mats, and picks up the blue-handled lawn mower, not the white-handled one he had taken from Danial. He holds it high in the air, straight up as far as his arm can reach. With the lawn mower stretched up into the air, he starts to grunt, squirm, grit his teeth, and flap his other hand. He sways the lawn mower in the air in a very slow circle and stares up at it.

Danial rolls over towards this scene. Looking at Thomas, Danial reaches out and takes back the white-handled lawn mower near him. He pulls the white-handled lawn mower underneath him and rolls over in the opposite direction again. Thomas stares at the circles he makes in the air. Thomas gradually lowers the lawn mower, laughing and gritting his teeth. He rests with the lawn mower to his side.

After a pause, the play resumes. Thomas again challenges Danial by raising the lawn mower over his head. It seems Danial does not want to play right now. He pushes his lawn mower over toward Thomas, who immediately withdraws the lawn mower from over Danial's head.

At this point the attendant enters and separates the two. The attendant looks and asks them, "What are you fighting for?" Moving the boys and dropping the toys sets the stage for continuing interaction, although this intervention is not directed, planned, or programmed. What is interpreted by the attendant as a fight is cooperative play.

For the time being, Danial seems to find the warmth of the sunlight more interesting than the toys or Thomas. He turns to the wall. Thomas wants to play. His persistence in the face of separation is admirable. As soon as he is on the mat, he moves into the aisle and picks up the blue-handled lawn mower (the original one he held). He holds it up in the air. Danial does not react until he suddenly rolls over. Perhaps the sound of Thomas's gritting teeth and his grunting require his attention. He recovers the white-handled lawn mower, puts it underneath him, and returns to rest. Thomas continues to swing the lawn mower.

Thomas moves closer to Danial. Again, they are parallel to one another, separated by a distance of four feet. Their positions are symmetrical so that when they come closer, their legs do not obstruct their contact with one another. Danial's legs are bent at the knees behind him like a jack-knife. Thomas's legs are also bent at the knees in front of him. As they approach each other, their positions complement each other.

An attendant brings in an aluminum chair to sit next to my lounge chair, right behind the two boys. She looks at the two boys near her but stays for only a short time. She gets up and walks through the sleeping area into the office. Danial has apparently fallen asleep. He lies quietly, snoring occasionally. Thomas looks at him once in a while, then away. He lies quietly or gives the lawn mower a few haphazard pushes and pulls.

Thomas initiates the third exchange. Dropping the blue-handled lawn mower, he reaches for the white-handled one under Danial. The handle is under Danial's waist and the lawn mower's cylinder protrudes behind his back.

Thomas slides his hand up and over the cylinder and up onto the handle. His hand moves halfway up the exposed handle and pulls it from underneath the sleeping body of Danial. He moves the handle down and towards himself, sliding his fist up the handle until about four inches from the cylinder. He holds the toy like a mallet now. He cocks, bringing the toy and his arm from the elbow back over his head. With his arm completely extended, he swings the lawn mower towards Danial. It falls short by a few inches. Because of the momentum of the swing, the lawn mower moves down past Thomas's legs. He allows it to fall loosely through his hand as it swings so that the toy falls the length of his arm and the length of the three-foot handle. His fingers grasp the tip of the handle before it flies out of reach. He grits his teeth, and gradually inches his way down the handle, passing the handle halfway through his fingers. He brings his hand up past his waist. He cocks his arm again. He pauses briefly, grits his teeth, and lets fly. Lawn mower and hand sweep the floor above and in front of him, in a wide arc. The momentum of the toy picks up as Thomas's grasp loosens on the handle. As he has moved his hand three quarters of the way down the handle, the trajectory seems to be on a collision course with the sleeper, but it falls short a second time.

Thomas grits his teeth. He wheels in the lawn mower once again, using the same slow, deliberate movements of the fingers as in his previous attempt. The gritting stops as he repositions himself by moving his whole body, not closer to Danial, but to improve the angle of his swing. He cocks his arm and hits again at Danial. He misses. His face stiffens and he immediately grits his teeth until he positions himself again, aims and fires. He hits his mark and on impact with Danial's back begins to hum. No reaction. Thomas repeats this entire sequence three times, each with varying degrees of contact. Twice the body of the lawn mower lands squarely on Danial; the third time it just brushes him, but with no reaction.

Thomas switches the position of the lawn mower to use the handle to poke Danial between his shoulder blades. No response. He switches the lawn mower again to use as a mallet and hits Danial on the shoulder. He switches to the left hand, and resumes the attack in the same characteristic fashion, this time hitting the elbow of the arm Danial has tucked under him. He lets fly another swing and misses. He grits his teeth once more. Rather than taking the toy back over his head, he nudges it against different points on Danial's back, moving up and down the right side of his back against the floor. Finally, he resumes the original position and hits Danial's back twice more, a third and final time.

As Thomas's provocation of Danial unfolds, an attendant sits down in the chair placed there by her predecessor (who stayed only during the beginning of the exchange). Thomas and Danial are almost right in front of her in the shadow of the chair. She peers out over the area.

In a surprise move, Danial rolls completely over on his stomach all at once. He lands on the blue handle of the lawn mower left in the aisle while Thomas pokes and hits Danial with the white-handled one. Thomas lets the white-handled toy drop beside him. Danial reaches toward the white-handled lawn mower while he is still recovering from his roll. He grabs it, picks it up and holds it in the air. He swings it in the air over Thomas and drops it on Thomas. Thomas grips the chair leg, pulling himself up and, placing his weight on his elbow, looks up and beyond Danial in the direction of the other lawn mower.

The attendant, who has been sitting in the chair only a few minutes, bends over and looks down at Danial. Without saying a word, she gets out of the chair, lifts it, and walks out into the sleeping area.

Thomas collapses to the floor as soon as he sees the attendant look down at him. He releases the chair leg and lies still as the chair moves over him. After the attendant's departure, he moves toward Danial, grabs the blue-handled lawn mower and pushes it onto Danial. With the jiggling of the handle under him, Danial reaches down to the handle, pulls it out from under him. He rolls over to get closer to Thomas. Rolling over, he bumps his head on the floor in the process, with a resounding crack. Danial pulls the blue-handled lawn mower completely out of Thomas's reach and turns over completely to Thomas. In position, he pushes the blue-handled lawn mower out towards Thomas. Thomas watches, but does not move. Danial again moves it out and back.

The attendant who left a few minutes earlier returns and asks the attendant who first sat in the chair (now in the middle of the activity room), "Can I put my shoes over there next to Danial?" She continues, "Danial, don't you get at them and throw them."

Danial watches as she leans over him to place her shoes down. At the same time, Thomas takes the white-handled lawn mower, and cocks his arm to aim at Danial. He lets go; Danial looks around to see the object coming toward him and throws the blue-handled toy towards Thomas, enough to cause Thomas's lawn mower to miss the mark. Thomas, tensing all of his muscles and gritting his teeth, places one foot against the floor. Pushing off with his hand, he raises his stiffened body like an arch over the floor with tremendous exertion. With one hand pushing, his head and his feet on the ground, he raises his mid-section into the air. With one more strain he pushes his body over the threshold and he falls on his stomach quickly to the ground with a dull thud. Humming, with a smile on his face, he moves himself toward Danial, his legs dragging behind. He heads toward the blue-handled lawn mower.

Finally, Thomas attempts to wake and engage Danial. Danial turns away from the action but also accepts Thomas's invitation. After rolling away from the activity and the action, he rolls back into it.

Thomas apparently rouses Danial. Danial rolls over, grabs the white-handled lawn mower, and drops it on Thomas. Thomas pulls himself up by the leg of the chair in which the attendant sits. She ignores the event. As she departs, Thomas retreats from the encounter. With her departure, Thomas lifts himself into position to retrieve the lawn mower. Lying facing Thomas, Danial once more places the lawn mower in the space between them. Danial does not arrange the activity to his own advantage, but impartially places the lawn mower in the middle. He competes fairly.

When Danial looks at the shoes, Thomas seizes the white-handled lawn mower and uses it as a mallet once again. The distraction works to Thomas's advantage. Surprised by the object being thrown at him, Danial turns over spontaneously and throws the blue-handled lawn mower toward Thomas. It misses. Thomas rolls closer, heads toward the blue-handled lawn mower and retrieves it.

After throwing the blue-handled lawn mower at Thomas, Danial rolls over away from the scene to face the wall. But as Thomas moves toward the lawn mower thrown at him, Danial turns completely over again to face Thomas and to recover the blue-handled lawn mower. Thomas reaches it first and pulls it towards him. Thomas also grabs the white-handled lawn mower. He strains to arch his body with great effort, falls away from Danial with the lawn mowers on the opposite side from Danial. With Danial staring at him, Thomas lies back and laughs out loud.

Two attendants coming on duty for the new shift enter from the bedroom area. Without a word, they pick up Thomas. One holds his head and the other his legs at the knees. He continues to laugh as they move him into the sleeping area. He grabs at the lawn mower, but it slides out of his hand as he is lifted.

Danial turns back over and towards the shoes that the attendant leaves on the floor. The attendant who places the shoes there asks the one seated in the center of the room to place them on the sill away from Danial. Danial looks around for a moment and then lies quietly on the floor. Thomas's laughter can still be heard from the sleeping area.

In the final sequence of the event, Danial rolls completely over in the opposite direction, toward the wall, but keeps the position for only a moment. Then he faces Thomas. Thomas recovers the blue-handled lawn mower and the white-handled one. Having secured both, he rolls over to set himself between the toys and Danial and laughs. Thomas is successful in capturing both toys. The play is interrupted because the attendants come in and remove Thomas. The lawn mowers fall across each other. Danial lies quietly, staring at them. Thomas laughs uproariously while being removed to the sleeping area.

The sequence in the play event is interrupted when the two attendants move Thomas from the activity area into the sleeping area. Thomas's laughter expresses his acknowledgement and appreciation of the play. In the end, he has both lawn mowers.

Summary

The play event is a sequence of interaction and interchange that is built over time. It follows a pattern mutually determined between the two individuals. They accommodate one another in their actions and reactions. The pattern in their movement and positioning includes repeated attempts to position themselves in such a way to allow the exchange of a toy.

Initially, the two boys arrange themselves compatibly and their physical arrangement allows the play event to proceed. The toy is the object of exchange and symbolic of their communication. The direct care staff are aware of the boys' interest in the toy and provide it without a second thought. Nor do they consider the toy important when they separate the boys. Danial and Thomas use the toy in a variety of ways. The toy has value as a medium for exchange, and as an extension of themselves – for example, to hit the doll, or to provoke action by prodding one another. Both boys travel great distances to recover the toy, and will roll over and position themselves to take turns. The example reveals deftness and calculation in their actions and shows their ability to plan movement and respond spontaneously to the other.

Summary

The residents choose whether or not to participate, pausing, for instance, to consider the other's situation and the presentation of challenges. In other examples, the residents collect their toys, visit their neighbors, initiate play and respond to a peer's plight. Danial and Thomas play to express their feelings for one another and they demonstrate purpose in overcoming obstacles to pursue their goal.

The patterns in their actions that evolve over two-and-a-half hours reveal the significance in the event. Motivation and incentive are sustained; the physical exertion necessary to travel great distances to play is maintained by both boys. No one segment or sequence in the event reveals its significance and meaning in isolation. While their behavioral repertoire is richer and fuller than any one individual behavior, attention to individual behaviors is a starting place to understand their actions. The differential use of a repertoire of response and interaction reveals the resilience, the versatility, and the exercise of will in their action.

Adopting the perspective of the residents reveals revised spatial and temporal aspects to their interaction with each other. Their behaviors are activated slowly and meticulously at their own pace. This does not mean that they do not act quickly. They react immediately to the presence of the attendant by stopping their own movements; they quickly grab the object the other has, or move out of its way. Danial and Thomas live in the entire space of the apartment, not just within the restrictions of the mat and its immediate surrounds. The distances they travel reveal their attention to different contexts.

It is the shared and learned aspects in the patterns of Danial's and Thomas's interaction that are significant. Both boys interpret the behavior and the expression of the other. They work out ways to play in the apartment. They avoid staff intervention – for example, separation. They respect one another's ability to participate yet continue to challenge one another in the context of their play.

The residents are a remarkably heterogeneous and complex group of individuals who demonstrate a wide range of ability and talent in their involvements with one another. Each responds in his own manner to the care and handling received in the context of events in the apartment. Left on their own, they attend to what goes on around them and what happens to them. The contours of individual pathology and the effect of pathology on functioning are realistic limits but do not represent all that they can do.

Howe emphasizes that "Nature produces individuals not classes." The play event between Danial and Thomas shows them to be individuals who have learned to share and participate in the context of their lives together. They demonstrate non-verbal language in gestures, vocalizations, and actions.

The model relating pathological condition to functional characteristics is the basis for interpreting the significance of the behavior in the play event. Danial and Thomas share more than the clinical description of their pathological condition. They share the richness of their ability to participate on their own in play, the complexity of their involvement and execution of movements and behaviors, and the simple enjoyment inherent in the activities and events when they engage each other. Given the constraints of their disability, they arrange themselves in this event so as to make it possible for one another to participate. The exchange of the toy is symbolic of their ability to make meaning in the course of living with each other. It is the shared meaning which accomplishes the exchange of the toy. In this example, each demonstrates expression – to use Howe's term – and each can understand and act in a social context. Their expressions have meaning and they act on the meaning conveyed. They demonstrate the full breadth of human contact within the constraints of their handicaps and the environment in which they live.

The context of the interaction or event determines its social meaning. The message contained within a behavior, its signal or sign, can be understood through a consideration of context. "Social" simply means what the residents do with one another when left to themselves. The residents' social life develops through their past and present experiences with other residents in and out of the classroom and primarily in the apartment. The social ability in this setting depends on the ability to understand the other residents but also the context of the event – for example, what staff permit. Chapter 4 identifies the dramatic impact which staff intervention has on the social behavior of the residents.

4

Residents' participation in programs

The historical context

Having conducted a study to determine the number and the condition of the feebleminded in the state of Massachusetts, Samuel G. Howe gained public support for the first permanent public school, the Massachusetts School for Idiotic and Feebleminded Youth, established on October 1, 1856.

The school was located within the community because Howe did not believe the feebleminded should be removed and segregated from a neighborhood community. He selected students on the basis of their potential for improvement and ability to benefit from instruction. The criterion for selection was Howe's definition of idiocy.

Idiocy is the condition of a human being in which, owing to some morbid cause in the bodily organization, the faculties and sentiments remain dormant or undeveloped, so that the person is incapable of self guidance, and of approaching that degree of knowledge usual with others of his age. (Howe, 1876:21)

Appropriate selection and classification were essential to justify the expenditure of funds. Howe stated that the most suitable idiots for instruction were those who enjoyed good bodily health, were not epileptic, and were without an enlarged head (Howe, 1853:12). The optimum age for the 5 to 7 years of schooling required for the feebleminded was from 7 years to 16 years of age. Their distinguishing feature was the presence of speech. Without the *habit* of speech, the individual lacked the distinguishing characteristic of man.

In the face of mounting pressure to admit increasing numbers of individuals and custodial cases, Howe tried to preserve his vision of a school for the feebleminded, and steadfastly maintained the position that the school should not become an asylum. He warned:

Now, the danger of misdirection in this pious and benevolent work is that two false principles may be incorporated into the projected institutions, which will be as rotten piles in the foundations, and make the future establishments deplorably defective and mischievous. These are, first, the close congregation; and second, the lifelong association of a large number of idiots; whereas, the true, sound principles are: *separation of idiots from each other; and the diffusion among the normal population.* The same thing applies to institutions for other classes of defectives and of dependents.

Even more than the lunatics, the very idea of life-asylums for idiots suggests, to thinking persons, formidable objections and grave consequences. It implies social and moral isolation and ostracism. It implies a sundering of the tender ties of family, and the important ties of neighborhood, with consequent loss of advantages, to the unfortunates, of observing and imitating normal people. It implies privation of the elevating influence of sane and superior associates. It implies lifelong companionship among those who act and re-act injuriously upon each other. For these and other reasons, it is unwise to organize establishments for teaching and training idiotic children, upon such principles as will make them tend to become asylums for life. (Howe, 1875:22–23)

Recognition of the problems faced by the feebleminded and their families and the growing need for services for the custodial cases led to the establishment of lifelong protective care for individuals unable to return to the community, and the extension of custodial care to improvable low-grade individuals in need of total care.

Howe's statements on the placement of the first public school for the mentally retarded recommended locating the school within the community in close proximity to the family. As the number of feebleminded continued to increase as a result of the growing commitment to the education and care of the feebleminded, Howe's school expanded; pressure increased to educate more and more individuals, provisions for lower and lower grades of idiocy were advocated, and the notion of lifelong care was promoted. Schools became asylums; asylums became farm colonies; farm colonies became institutions; institutions became training schools; and training schools have decreased in number in recent years as a return to the community has been advocated.

Custodial care was a new development in the care of the feebleminded in the United States in the late 1800s. The admittance of low-grade custodial cases represented a significant shift in the development of institutional care. The precedent for custodial care was the extension of lifetime protective care to individuals unable to return to their families or maintain themselves in the community. The first initiative taken in the introduction of custodial care was to occupy and maintain adults in farm colonies. This precedent set the stage for a second shift: the admittance at a very young age of low-grade custodial individuals for whom the potential for education and development was thought minimal but who, it was believed, had every right to protection and care.

The study of families of individuals who were feebleminded was begun in earnest in an effort to trace the inherited trait of feeblemindedness

(Dugdale 1877; Rogers and Merrill 1919; Winship 1900). Goddard sought to perform such a "natural experiment": the following summary describes his findings of the Kallikak family from the state of New Jersey.

We find on the good side of the family (Kallikaks) prominent people in all walks of life and nearly all of the 494 descendants owners of land or proprietors. On the bad side we find paupers, criminals, prostitutes, drunkards, and examples of all forms of social pests with which modern society is burdened.

From this we conclude that feeblemindedness is largely responsible for these social sores.

Feeblemindedness is hereditary and transmitted as surely as any other character. We cannot successfully cope with these conditions until we recognize feeblemindedness and its hereditary nature, we recognize it early, and take care of it.

In considering the question of care, segregation through colonization seems in the present state of our knowledge to be an ideally and perfectly satisfactory method. Sterilization may be accepted as a makeshift, as a help to solve this problem because the conditions have become so intolerable. But this must at present be regarded only as a makeshift and temporary, for before it can be extensively practiced, a great deal must be learned about the effects of the operation and about the laws of human inheritance. (Goddard, 1912:117)

Deborah Kallikak was one member of the Kallikak family so isolated (Doll 1983:30–32). At the time of Deborah's admittance to the institution for the mentally retarded, the care and education were doctrinaire. The resident moved within a scheduled system, arranged on the basis of expectations for her accomplishments in life. Selection for training on skills and tasks was determined by the individual's performance under the supervision of the staff. The resident was trained in the occupations of the institution. Decisions were based, in part, on scientific knowledge of what the feebleminded of a certain degree of idiocy, and of a particular mental and chronological age, could accomplish. Belief in innate capacity as measured by the intelligence test did much to determine the expectations of professionals and educators working with the feebleminded.

As experience within the institution confirmed these expectations about an individual resident, the educational goals and objectives for those with a similar degree or level of retardation were fixed. A confidence and self-assuredness about what was being done for the feebleminded developed in this period of institutionalization. Mental measurement confirmed this confidence. Positivism in setting educational goals within the institution developed as an extension of the scientific knowledge of medicine, psychology, and research of the time.

While the scientific accuracy assisted in the identification and selection of individuals within the institution, provision for the education and care of the severely and profoundly mentally retarded and multiply handicapped was to await legislation. Of the custodial area little is known, except for the description provided by Fernald of initial glimpses into the every day life of these residents. While institutional conditions were studied, systematic inquiry into the nature of care and treatment was to await the professional involvement of the 1970s. Up to this period, the severely and profoundly mentally retarded and multiply handicapped in this setting on the whole received basic care, with provisions for needs defined in terms of activities of daily living.

The legislative initiatives in relation to the mentally retarded and the handicapped in the last decade provided a framework for the provision of services to the severely and profoundly mentally retarded and multiply handicapped (Cohen and DeYoung, 1973). Such initiatives have radically changed the services provided to the handicapped in both scope and number. Early court decisions extended equal civil rights and due process: in Brown v. Board of Education (1954), the United States Supreme Court set the stage for equal educational opportunity for the handicapped; Hobsen v. Hansen (1967, 1971) abolished tracking of individuals into programs; Diana v. Board of Education (1970) prevented assessment of ethnic groups with culturally biased tests and raised the issues of the appropriateness of testing. Pennsylvania Association for Retarded Children v. Commonwealth of Pennsylvania (1971) established the right of education of the mentally retarded in the public schools; Mills v. Board of Education of the District of Columbia (1971) secured the right to instruction and training for the handicapped. Rights were extended in specific cases to institutionalized handicapped in residential facilities (New York State Association for Retarded Children, Inc. v. Rockefeller 1972; Ricci v. Greenblatt 1972, in Massachusetts; Wyatt v. Stickney 1971, 1972a, 1972b in Alabama) to prevent inhumane conditions, overcrowding, understaffing, servitude, and the lack of rehabilitation programming.

These court decisions hastened state regulations to provide a full range of services to individuals in a flexible manner in all cities and towns – for example Massachusetts Acts 1972: Chapter 766, "An Act ... Regulating Programs for Children Requiring Special Education" – the state was to set up regional advisory agencies and to provide programs for the handicapped as well as programs for professional development and training. Federal legislation and Executive Orders of the President stated that no agency or institution receiving federal funds could discriminate against the handicapped (Ford, 1976). These acts insured access for the handicapped to public buildings, jobs, and training.

The culmination of state legislation and court decisions was a federal statute, "Education of the Handicapped Act," enacted in 1975. The time line for provision of public education and services for all handicapped individuals under the legislation (ages 3–18) was September 1978 and for all individuals with handicaps (ages 3–21), not later than September 1980. It provided the cornerstone for present practice with the provision of free, appropriate special education services based on an individualized educational program in the least restrictive environment.

In the institutions, administrators and staff struggled to interpret the legislation, act judicially on behalf of the residents, and improve programs and buildings to satisfy the requirement for funding. State and federal inspections and court monitoring resulted in changes throughout the institutions. Controversies over the definitions of "free," "appropriate," and "least restrictive" were decided in the courts as staff sought their own interpretation and definitions. Controversies and the shifts in interpretations complicated the process of implementation.

In yet another domain, the 1971 Amendments to Title XIX of the Social Security Act (1965) allocated funds to develop new facilities and improve existing conditions and expanded Medicaid coverage to the long-term care of the disabled in mental institutions and nursing homes. Although funds were directed to bring institutions into line with federal standards, this act was criticized for encouraging an outdated model of institutional care and services, rather than providing support of programs and facilities within the community (Taylor *et al.*, 1981).

Three popular concepts in health care and human services emerged: deinstitutionalization, mainstreaming, and normalization. The isolated, backward custodial cases of Fernald's time were now the target of mandated services and experienced in their daily life the effects of current debate of these concepts by professionals. As residents of greater ability moved into the community, the question arose of how to apply the concepts of mainstreaming, normalization, and deinstitutionalization to the severely and profoundly mentally retarded and multiply handicapped who remained.

Howe's warnings forecast what was to occur with the development of institutions throughout the early 1900s – that is, the congregation and lifelong association of residents within the institution. Initially, the population was separated within the institution by degree and type of feeblemindedness. The process of clinical classification led to the assignment of specific buildings and wards within institutions. Howe's statements remind us that thought on placement of the mentally retarded has come full circle. The concepts of deinstitutionalization, mainstreaming, and normalization provide the more recent conceptualizations and guide current practice. They represent a return to original notions and concepts about where the education and care of the feebleminded should take place. In this setting, these terms are used repeatedly to justify the goals, objectives and philosophy of the program, and the aim toward which professional practice is directed. That is, deinstitutionalization seeks to provide alternative, community-based services and residences for the developmentally disabled. Mainstreaming advocates the education of handicapped individuals within the least restrictive environment with other students of the same age and grade. Normalization requires the provision for participation in the natural and everyday human interaction within a society and culture. These are concepts based on attempts to realign the relationship of the residents inside the institution with the experience of others outside the institution – the mainstream of society.

"Normal" for the residents

Institutional care and treatment, once thought to be innovative and appropriate, has been problematic in its impersonality; deinstitutionalization advocates a return to the community (Paul *et al.*, 1977). The concept of deinstitutionalization represents a role change for the institution:

Deinstitutionalization encompasses three interrelated processes: (1) prevention of admission by finding and developing alternative methods of care and training; (2) return to the community of all residents who have been prepared through programs of habilitation and training to function adequately in appropriate local settings; and (3) establishment and maintenance of a responsive residential environment which protects human and civil rights and which contributes to the expeditious return of the individual to normal community living, whenever possible. (National Association of Superintendents of Public Residential Facilities for the Mentally Retarded, 1974)

This definition is consistent with the development of a range of services for the handicapped. It implies that the institution represents the most restrictive form of placement and should be reserved for those individuals for whom other alternatives are not feasible. A policy of deinstitutionalization involves the placement of residents into programs and services within the community and, for those who remain in the institution, increased participation in community programs. Deinstitutionalization represents a change in setting, location and relation to mainstream society and culture which is designed to provide the opportunity for normal interaction and participation.

If we view deinstitutionalization from the perspective of the residents, however, the question arises whether we fully appreciate the nature of their communicative and interactive difference or understand the ways in which we must interact with them to normalize the interaction for them. Advocacy of deinstitutionalization implies removal of residents from institutions to minimize the negative effect of living in the institution. The decision to release an individual from an institution is a complex one,

involving consideration of the requirements for preparation, reintegration, and resocialization into society, community, and the family.
Consideration must also be given to the relationships among programs
and agencies and to the individual rights of access in the community (Paul
et al., 1977).

The concept of mainstreaming – the integration of handicapped individuals into regular or mainstream living and learning environments –
implies a homogeneous definition of what is normal, regular, and appropriate. Integration into the regular classroom has been facilitated through
a graded series of programs, learning activities and experiences to achieve
acculturation.

In the definition provided by the Council for Exceptional Children
(1975:74) mainstreaming is:

providing the most appropriate education for each child in the least
    restrictive setting
looking at the educational needs of children instead of clinical or
    diagnostic labels...
looking for and creating alternatives that will help general educators serve
    children with learning or adjustment problems in the regular setting...
uniting the skills of general education and special education so all children
    may have equal educational opportunity.

Mainstreaming is not:

wholesale return of all exceptional children in special classes to regular
    classes
permitting children with special needs to remain in regular classrooms
    without support services that they need
ignoring the need of some children for a more specialized program than
    can be provided in the general education program
less costly than servicing children in special self-contained classrooms.

This viewpoint seems to be closer to the mainstream and it assumes a
mainstream cultural reference point – that is, the degree to which
programs in the regular classroom are less restrictive. The difficulty arises
when individual ability and settings are assessed from the perspective of
how closely they approximate "normal conditions." The emphasis is on
the assessment of the individual's ability to interact and participate in the
normal learning environment, rather than maintaining the interactional
style and contexts which allow the individual to participate in a manner
consistent with their evolved ways of interacting with others.

Normalization becomes a criterion by which to judge the setting, the
program, and the individual. Idealized as a process and a goal, a corrective
principle for programming, and an ideology, normalization is the direct

113

application of standards, conventions, and etiquette from the mainstream to the severely and profoundly mentally retarded. Normalization assumes that behaviors can be shaped to match those of a normal individual of the same age and sex; it implies structuring of a way of life to minimize the fact, the appearance, and the effect of deviancy:

Utilization of means which are as culturally normative as possible, in order to establish and maintain personal behaviors and characteristics which are as culturally normative as possible...

[Normalization implies] that in as many aspects of a person's functioning as possible, the human manager will aspire to elicit and maintain behaviors and appearances that come as close to being normative as circumstances and the person's behavioral potential permit. (Wolfensberger, 1972:28)

Wolfensberg goes on to advocate the arrangement, type, and quality of facilities, programs, and behaviors based on "normal" *appearances*.

But the goal of homogeneity is as spurious for the mainstream as it is for the mentally retarded, for normalization is a stereotype based on appearances. That the individual can look and act like his peers is an assumption. If the actions of the severely and profoundly mentally retarded can be understood as a consequence of their desires, wants, and needs, caretakers and professionals must accept the challenge of understanding their world and the significance of their choices, and must respect their differences. But understanding the differences in the condition of the severely and profoundly mentally retarded and multiply handicapped and its impact on the individual is essential to a redefinition of the ways in which they are "normal." The choices which they make themselves are relevant to the differences in their experience and involvement with each other.

Wolfensberger (1972) advocates choice for individuals within institutions:

Normalization also dictates that a person should be as independent, free to move about, and empowered to make meaningful choices as are typical citizens of comparable age in the community. As much as possible, his wishes and desires should carry the same weight as they would in ordinary circumstances outside of a human management context. (p. 87)

But decisions about "normalizing experiences" for the severely and profoundly mentally retarded and multiply handicapped can only really be evaluated from the perspective and within the context of the life experience of the individuals themselves.

The concepts of mainstreaming, normalization, and deinstitutionalization are ways to articulate the goals and processes of professional intervention. The concepts in themselves do not entail any change in perspective to examine what the severely and profoundly mentally retarded do, but instead involve placing them into programs to facilitate acculturation. The concepts are ways of explaining existing programs – a basis on which to structure and organize services at the program level – and they reflect a mainstream perspective. These concepts can in practice militate against the interests of the individual who is severely and profoundly mentally retarded and multiply handicapped. Applying the concept of normalization to the care and treatment of the severely and profoundly mentally retarded, however well-intentioned, advocates change in the alignment of programs and services inside and outside the institution. However, care and treatment should begin not just with reconceptualization or reorganization of programs and services and models, but rather with understanding how those programs and services can assist the severely and profoundly mentally retarded in the development of their natural ability. Clearly delineating their demonstrated competencies respects first what they do, before interventions are determined and programs changed. The institutional daily schedule, the services, and the programs for the residents need to be finely tuned to the understanding of the residents' individual differences. Systematic inquiry into their life experience to determine its rhythm, tempo, sound, movement, and pattern is one form of interpretation.

Programs developed on the basis of the popular concepts of mainstreaming, normalization, and deinstitutionalization, will be incomplete unless we have first attempted to understand the life of the severely and profoundly mentally retarded. A cultural interpretation of their action would regard "normality" as what is normal for the severely and profoundly mentally retarded, given the nature of their differences.

Resident programs

This chapter contrasts what the residents do on their own, exemplified in the play of Danial and Thomas, with their interaction with professional staff during programmed activities. This discussion of the differences in performance highlights the fact that the residents perform differently on their own from the way they behave with professionals.

Professional knowledge about what the residents do is the basis for intervention. Different professional disciplines generate information about pathology and functioning but integrate that information in different ways, on the basis of the discipline itself and the ability of the individual professional. The doctor has a commitment to understanding the clinical condition as a primary emphasis. The physical therapist understands the clinical condition and functioning in a specific area of performance. The educator has a commitment to performance regardless of the clinical condition across all areas of development.

Thus concepts which guide professional practice must be carefully scrutinized for their relation to what the resident actually does. History shows that residents have continually been subject to changes in conceptualization of what is appropriate for them. Because our knowledge is based primarily on clinical analysis of their behavior and understanding of the clinical characteristics of their condition, it is primarily an understanding of the handicapping condition rather than of the individual's performance within the constraints of the handicap. The residents' participation is relative to the nature of their disability, their ability to exercise control over the competing demands of their pathological condition, their understanding of the situation and the interactional demands, and their ability to initiate or respond within the framework of the other interactants.

In this setting, the inauguration of educational and therapeutic programs represents the fullest extension of professional practice to this population within the institution in a comprehensive and systematic form (1979–80). The examples describe the experience of Danial and Thomas in their first year of full participation in programs structured and organized to meet their individual needs. The difference in styles of interaction and participation in the lesson is viewed in terms not of the presence or absence of ability, but rather in terms of the social and cultural characteristics of interaction and participation. The irony in the examples is that Danial's and Thomas's interaction is not understood for what it is – that is, their ability to read the context of the lesson and the choices they make about participation.

The cornerstone of professional practice in this setting is the process of clinical assessment and determination of the skills and abilities of the resident. Each resident is subject to the same process of clinical scrutiny. The uniformity of the process and the conformity of professionals to the application of the clinical model produce a remarkably similar set of descriptions and explanations for behavior and performance. With a highly heterogeneous population, the approach is homogenized into a description of sets of skills and abilities. Within the setting, a uniform procedure has evolved for the examination, analysis, and recording of resident behavior. The environment complies with health and safety standards and with the amount of privacy and individual space deemed appropriate in a group living situation. Apartment rules of management keep the residents on the mats and their toys out of the aisles. The examples over the years of this study show an increasing proliferation of programs and activities based on a uniform set of procedures, mainstream assumptions, a normative order to skill development, and communication in reports and among staff which obscure the reality of the residents' performance in an interaction. The examples in this chapter make a case for attending to the meaning implicit in the diversity and difference of the residents' responses to their daily life. Understanding their differences makes plain the need to change the patterns explicit in our interaction with them. Understanding the patterns in their behavior is the starting point for our participation with them.

This study began prior to inauguration of a fully organized and structured program (1978) and traced the development and the implementation of the programs and the subsequent effects on the residents' daily lives in the second period of the observation (1979–80). During the first period of observation (January–June 1978) the residents participated in activities which related to basic care and attention to their medical and health needs. The example of Danial and Thomas in chapter 3 shows the two residents in play over an extended period of time. The example reveals the mutual nature of their repertoires of behavior in patterns of play together – for instance, pausing to consider the other's situation and presentation of challenges to one another. In 1978, the residents interacted with one another despite their numbers. In retrospect, the number of individuals on the mats increased the opportunity for interaction: supervision focused on preventing accidents and changing diapers, and residents were left on their own much of the time.

The second period of observation (1979–80) saw the refinement of programs, the implementation of diagnostic assessment and the annual review of individualized educational plans. In addition to observing behavior, collecting data, and implementing and conducting resident programs, the professional staff supervise lessons by teacher-aides, volunteers, and parents. The residents participate in structured interactions with the staff, or have formal contacts which arise out of the professional staff fulfilling their responsibilities, for most of the day.

In 1980, the two boys' play interaction recalled the richness and fullness of their accomplishment observed in 1978 (see chapter 3). In the interval, the context of the activity area had changed. During the rest period, residents were now separated on the mats by greater distances. The residents now interacted less when they were together on their own, and they slept more. With the elimination of the morning and the afternoon activity periods in the apartment, they had fewer long stretches of time together.

The social dimensions of the residents' lives, exemplified by the case of Danial and Thomas, are revealing. The professionals are developing the residents' social behavior through developmental steps of functional skills. Because the skills are viewed as linear, the solution to development is to switch back and forth, up and down the ladder of skills to find one the resident can perform.

However, the residents develop their social skills primarily in the apartment, in interactions with others. The residents learn to understand context, the meaning of events, the function of personnel, and the plan and order of the day's activities. With limited awareness of demonstrated skills of social interaction such as those of Danial and Thomas, the teachers program social skill development below or outside the range of the residents' ability. Since the medium for intervention is the diagnostic prescriptive process, failure in the lesson leads to evaluation of the task and discussion of what the resident does and does not do. Failure in the lesson does not lead to observation of *social* situations in which Danial and Thomas participate.

One result of program development and scheduling is that interaction of the residents is restricted primarily to staff. The social context to interaction is defined in terms of staff, not residents. Residents have less opportunity to be involved with each other in the naturally occurring events which are fundamental to their social fabric; the basis of their life together is disrupted more and more by the institutionalized process of individualized instruction.

Differences in the attendants' and the volunteers' approaches to the residents are also evident. The staff interactions become formalized – that is, formulas determine what is to be said and done. The direct care staff repeat these formulas and expressions in the presence of the professional staff and defer to them during interactions with a resident. Direct care staff withdraw from their own sense of knowing and their own spontaneous interaction in the belief that the professional staff know more, thus distancing themselves from the residents and from the responsibility of providing anything more than direct care.

In 1978, the attendants were able to observe the lessons of the teachers and the play activities of the residents, and were even able to participate in their development of patterns. The attendants in apartment A were fewer in number than in apartments M and N, but were more involved in the provision of daily care as an activity. They were continuously involved with the chores of the apartment from the early morning to the mid-afternoon shift change. In 1980, the attendants did not see the teachers and the professionals conduct their lessons and activities on the activity area, since the teachers and therapists all had classrooms, work areas and specially equipped rooms. The music therapist was the only individual who regularly visited the ward and conducted activities there. The archive records evidence the change. The attendants wrote less in the progress notes as the professional comments increased and grew more sophisticated. The direct care staff participated in the development of the individualized program to a lesser extent. Their relationship remained less formal and less encumbered with the particularities of the diagnostic prescriptive plan but was nevertheless individualized. They cared for the residents assigned to them for the day. In 1980 the attendants were more attentive to the guidelines, keeping the residents on the mats, and quiet during rest periods.

Resident programs

The following examples are from the second period of observation. They illustrate Danial's and Thomas's interaction in structured programs with staff. In the first example, Danial and Thomas interact and participate in the morning class with a teacher and a teacher aide and with fellow residents. In the second example a volunteer foster grandmother feeds Thomas at lunchtime. The rest period follows; it includes an examination and therapy with a physical therapist. Finally, an afternoon socialization class presents a lesson designed to teach Danial and Thomas peer socialization and play skills.

Morning classroom activity

The teachers, aides, and student teachers are involved in the feeding programs and prepare the residents for class by combing their hair. By 9:30, after breakfast, showers, dressing and hair-combing, they move the residents into individual classrooms for the morning activity period. This classroom is located in back of the sleeping area in the solarium. This leaves the activity area of the apartment vacant, except for those over 22 years who are no longer eligible for educational programming.

In the classroom are one teacher and two teacher aides. Today, a student teacher works in the classroom with one individual. The teachers, with the aides, construct lessons designed to teach a particular skill. The lessons have evolved from program priorities set for the resident at the annual review. In the classroom on this day are the following residents: Maxine, Joseph, May, Beverly, Barbara, Danial, and Thomas. The male teacher aide works with Thomas, Danial, and Joseph on the right side of the solarium, moving from one to the other in the course of the activity. The female teacher aide spends her time on the right side of the room with May, Barbara, and Beverly on the mats, cushions and triangular wedges. The teacher stands in the center of the room, overseeing all of the activities and rationing her time between Maxine, Barbara, and Beverly. On a table behind her rest charts and notebooks of resident programs.

Joseph sits and rolls his head against the back of the chair while the male teacher-aide works with Danial and Maxine. Maxine sits in her adapted wheelchair; the proximity of the wheelchair to the ground and its molded seat make it appear as if she sits in a stroller. In front of her is a board with pictures propped up from the Peabody Language Development Kit. In front of the board sits the male teacher-aide with a bell and a ball and Danial alongside him on the mat. The teacher-aide sits between them, telling Danial, "Look up at Maxine." When he does, the teacher-aide congratulates him with the expression, "Good boy." He then turns his attention to Maxine saying, "Look at Danial." She casts her eyes down and he exclaims, "Good girl." He then hands the ball to Danial telling him, "Take the ball. Roll it to Maxine." Danial looks up at the aide and down at the ball repeatedly. The aide repeats the directions. Danial then slowly pushes the ball with his left arm. Maxine watches the ball and smiles. The ball touches her wheelchair and the aide exclaims, "Good." He tells

Maxine to look at Danial and roll the ball to him. When she smiles and grows rigid, the aide taps the ball at the front of Maxine's wheelchair and pushes it over to Danial. The ball bounces up against Danial's chest. The aide repeats the sequence over and over and rings the bell when the ball rolls between them. Maxine smiles and sometimes coughs when the ball rolls away from the foot of her wheelchair toward Danial. She watches the ball roll the entire distance of two feet between them, grows rigid and smiles when Danial touches or moves the ball. The aide continues his exclamations, "Roll the ball!" and "Good boy!" and "Good girl!" sometimes saying to Maxine, "Danial is your boyfriend." Maxine continues to look at Danial as he turns over and away from the activity.

The teacher-aide then asks if Maxine would like to do the cards. Maxine nods her assent and smiles broadly. The aide tries to coax Danial back into the activity but cannot budge him. The aide gives him the ball and places Thomas on a mat opposite him. The two stare at each other and the ball remains motionless.

The aide checks Danial and Thomas. "Are you rolling the ball?" Neither has rolled the ball. He pushes the ball into the center and it sits there as he goes to Joseph.

After changing the record for Joseph and listening into the earphones, the teacher-aide turns his attention to Danial and Thomas. As they lie there motionless on the mat, the aide sits down at their head and says, "O.K., come on you two, pass the ball." He passes the ball between them but cannot get them to do the same. After prompting the interaction three times, he exclaims, "Do it or else I'm going to get mad." He tries once more to get them to pass the ball and says to the teacher, "Thomas is getting mad at me." The teacher suggests moving Thomas over to the inclined triangular wedge for the rest of the activity period to try positioning. The aide and the teacher pick him up and move him up to a wedge at the other end of the room. They position him in a prone position facing up the incline. The incline faces away from the wall and toys are placed out in front of him so that he has to lift his head and move his hands in front of him to play with the toys. The aide returns to Joseph, and the teacher returns to Beverly to rub her arms and her neck, talking to her quietly at the same time.

The male teacher aide takes the earphones off Joseph and swings the rocking chair in the opposite direction. He lifts him out of the chair and onto the mat in front of it. Danial rolls over and reaches for the frisbee lying on the mat. The aide says, "Want it? You better go the other way" (suggesting to Danial that he move in the opposite direction, not in the way of the aide working with Joseph). Danial smiles and turns over, holding the frisbee.

The teacher-aide sits between Danial and Maxine and directs their interaction. Typically, the teacher-aide follows a lesson designed by the teacher. The teacher identifies a behavioral response and its reward. For example, if Danial rolls the ball, the teacher-aide says, "Good boy!" In the example, the teacher-aide mediates each behavior. He rolls the ball for Maxine. After several repetitions of the direction, Danial complies and rolls the ball to Maxine. With the aid of the teacher, they repeat the sequence. Both Maxine and Danial acknowledge their participation in the activity. Maxine coughs and smiles when the ball rolls away from the wheelchair. She grows rigid and smiles when the ball reaches Danial. Danial continues to roll the ball. The teacher rings the bell and exclaims, "Good boy!" and "Good girl!" Suddenly, Danial rolls away and cannot be coaxed to return. As the teacher-aide returns his attention toward a new activity with Maxine, Danial and Thomas find themselves face-to-face (not head-to-toe as in the previous play example).

When the teacher-aide returns to the two boys they do not heed his request. The teacher-aide "threatens" them. Even if off the cuff, his remark seems out of place in this context. The aide announces his lack of success to the teacher but places the responsibility on Thomas and personalizes Thomas's reaction.

The teacher recommends changing the activity and switches the context. Thomas has no choice. In a new position on the wedge, Thomas must move in a different way to get the toys. Although its therapeutic value justifies this position, Thomas still does not play with the toys.

Danial lies still until he spots the frisbee. The teacher-aide suggests the way to get it. Having the frisbee gives Danial what he wants. As is the case for Thomas on the wedge, however, being near the toys is not the same as being in a position that facilitates the way he plays. Staring at the space in front of them, the boys await their turn with a teacher.

The aide now picks up a wooden box with different shapes cut in the four different sides and brings it over to Danial. "Come on, let's go," he says to Danial putting the box down beside him. He empties the box and the objects fall in front of Danial. "Come on Danial, put them in the box." While the shapes fit the holes cut in the sides of the box, the aide unlatches one whole side. Now they can just be placed into the box. The aide demonstrates and puts one shape into the box. He reaches for Danial's hand and tells him he will ring the bell every time he does it. "Come on Danial. Danial." The aide shakes the box. "Put them in the box. Come on, let's go. Let's go, come on." Danial is motionless. "Da...nial. Da...nial." Instead of picking up the objects to put in the box, Danial picks up the bell and puts it over his face. "Put it in the box." Danial puts the bell in the box. "Thank you." The teacher-aide rings the bell in the box. Danial laughs at the ring. The teacher aide takes the bell and rings it again and says, "Come on, put it in the box." Danial pushes away the box. The aide repeats three more times, "Put it in the box." The teacher, who looks over repeatedly, now listens to the aide's explanation of what is going on. "He doesn't want to work. Nobody likes me today." He looks down at Danial, "I'll give you play time when the session is over," he promises. Danial holds up his fist to the aide. "Don't give me the fist!" he exclaims. He pushes the box away and substitutes the ball saying, "O.K., come on, roll the ball." The aide sits in front of Danial for a few more seconds and then gets up to mark his chart.

Placing the different shapes into the holes in a box is a regularly scheduled activity. The aide initiates this activity without enthusiasm. The aide rearranges the purpose for which the box is designed and encourages Danial to place the shapes inside the large opening. The aide demonstrates the behavior and coaxes Danial. Instead Danial picks up the bell. The teacher accepts the change and rings the bell after Danial puts it in the box. The aide is frustrated when Danial does not continue. Danial chooses not to participate with the aide. The aide's persistence does not win Danial's cooperation. The teacher watches but offers no suggestions.

The female teacher-aide places a mirror in front of Thomas. Toys lie between Thomas and the mirror. The aide sits beside Thomas encouraging him to play with the toys, an assorted set of plastic dolls and shapes and animal figures. He is not allowed to touch the mirror, only to watch himself. The aide manipulates the objects saying, "See this one. Look at this. See yourself in the mirror." She tells the student teacher over her shoulder to follow what she is doing. They chat about the upcoming spring break and their plans. The aide shouts across the aisle to Barbara encouraging her to play with May. Because she appears so uncomfortable in the position in which she has been placed, May's smile seems produced to get attention rather than to express pleasure. "Hit the doll on the string," repeats the aide, interrupting the conversation about vacation. When the teacher takes Barbara off the mat, puts her in the wheelchair and brings her to the center of the room, the aide switches to work with Beverly. Working with her means picking her up off the mat, placing her between her legs and talking to her quietly, rubbing her back. This relaxation is in preparation for the lunchtime program of feeding.

The activity in the room comes to a stop.

"O.K., let's get them in their wheelchairs," says the teacher, watching Beverly. The social worker and student slip out the door. The two aides get up immediately to put the residents into their wheelchairs to move into the dining area. Danial is put in a stretcher and rolled halfway up the aisle of the sleeping area.

The aide working with Thomas is absorbed in her conversation about the upcoming vacation. Since she does not attend to Thomas, any meaningful response on his part is lost. Then it's time for lunch. This two hour morning classroom program places different demands on Danial's and Thomas's participation from those of the rest period in the activity area during the first period of observation (see chapter 3). The teacher's demands for interaction between the two boys follow a script of activities designed to teach a specific skill. Their participation in the lesson does not even mimic what they have done on their own. The lessons are organized to meet specific objectives. The two boys choose whether or not to participate, and they choose to participate in their own way, their own time and place.

Resident programs

Evaluation of performance on the objectives does not address the nature of their ability to participate, and may misrepresent what Danial and Thomas are really doing. Performance is measured from the point of view of what they don't do.

Lunchtime

To the far side of the dining area one grandmother feeds Thomas in about ten minutes. She grabs Thomas's stretcher bed and jerks it back up against the wall. Thomas cocks his head and looks over the back of the chair. He starts to grit his teeth loudly. The grandmother puts down her pocketbook on the chair and walks over to get his lunch. Returning to the chair, she positions herself at his side. Thomas reaches to grab her arm and turns away. He grits his teeth even louder. "Now stop that." She grabs both hands and puts them down by his side. She grabs his head and yanks it toward her. He grits his teeth all the louder. She takes up the bowl of food from the arm rest. Then in a systematic, continuous motion, she fills the spoon, puts it into his mouth, gets another spoon full, and repeats this until the bowl is empty (about three minutes). Thomas grunts as he eats, having time only to gulp the food. When she catches sight of one of the other grandmothers watching her she says, "Look what I had to do for him" (pointing to the bib she had to tie around his neck). She then gets up for the sherbert dessert and places it beside the bed stretcher so that he can see it. He looks and she says, "You like this don't you!" She takes up the spoon and shovels it into his mouth. She picks up the milk and drops it down his throat on the heels of the sherbert. He puts his tongue out through his lips as if to stop her but she continues to pour the milk into his mouth. In four continuous gulps, the milk is gone. Thomas grasps for air and breathes heavily. The grandmother wipes his mouth with the bib and brings the bowls over to the food cart. She then goes over to him and sits down beside him and looks at the others being fed (for twenty minutes).

Thomas is fed a bowl of food in three minutes, sherbert and milk in seven. Another grandmother looks at Thomas and says, "Want to take a walk?" and wheels him down the hall until rest period begins.

This lunchtime Thomas is not so lucky. The foster grandmother has demonstrated her displeasure about Thomas's behavior for the last few weeks. Thomas grits his teeth when he sees that she is there to feed him. He recognizes her and does not want to be fed by her. Thomas turns away, bending back over the chair, and grits his teeth in displeasure. He tries to grab her arm. On subsequent occasions he tries to grab her pocketbook, to scratch her, and keeps his mouth closed so that she cannot feed him. The feeding program becomes a test of wills. The foster grandmother shovels the food into his mouth, one spoonful after another. There is little Thomas can do if he wants to eat. For now, Thomas chooses to eat.

Residents' participation in programs

Rest period

The older male attendant rolls Thomas back in and places him on the mat in the center of the room. Thomas looks around and the attendant throws a pillow onto his chest. Thomas laughs.

Pamela and Maxine are on the water bed together. They do not look at each other. Barbara lies back on her triangular wedge and watches Thomas from across the room. Patrick is rolled out of the dining area and watches the movement of the wheelchairs back and forth as the residents are brought in and placed on the mat. Some come from the classroom, a few come from the cafeteria across the hall. The new attendant pulls May to the top of the wedge and gives her a hug. "How do you sleep down here?" he says with a smile. Danial, also thrown a pillow, rolls it over his face and vomits onto the pillow. He lies there quietly.

Dana lets out a scream. The same attendant who just quieted him yells over, "Oh, stop your screaming." She walks through to the Shower Area.

Thomas moves the pillow from his chest and crawls underneath a large piece of cardboard propped against the side wall of the divider over him. The cardboard forms a triangular tent over him.

During the rest period, a physical therapist comes in to talk to Thomas, lying on the mat. "Hi, Thomas." A nurse arrives from the opposite direction and says, "Hi, Thomas." They kneel down beside him and without another word, take off his shirt and pants. As she pulls off his shirt, the physical therapist says, "Come on, Thomas." She stretches the shirt over the coiled arm. The nurse undoes his pants and pulls them down around his bent knees.

Thomas starts to roll himself over and away from the nurse and the therapist. They both stare at him and his movement. Their eyes widen and their foreheads furrow as they watch. "He won't do that again."

They get up and move to his other side. He repeats the roll to the opposite side. They look at one another as they roll him back. After two attempts, he succeeds in making the roll in the direction opposite to them. The nurse moves to the side to which he has just rolled. The physical therapist moves to his head, with Thomas grunting and gritting his teeth. The physical therapist tries to hold his head and flex the muscles of his arm. Thomas rolls over away from her toward the nurse. This is the last time that he rolls away, although he makes one more attempt. The examination proceeds, with Thomas sandwiched in between the two professionals.

The only other movement he accomplishes is to turn his head away from them whenever they address him directly. The examination proceeds. The nurse rubs her hands over his chest and the physical therapist takes notes. The physical therapist takes his left, then his right arm and extends them as far as he can move them. Thomas pulls them back. The physical therapist stops when he resists. The nurse shakes a rattle in front of him. Thomas looks quickly and turns away. The physical therapist takes up his left arm, extends, rotates, and shakes it. Thomas moves up toward the physical therapist in the direction his arm is being pulled. She stops the extension, watching him move his legs and arms in the direction she is pulling.

Resident programs

The physical therapist takes up the rattle and again shakes it to either side in front of him. Thomas does not turn toward it this time at all. The physical therapist shakes the rattle on the left, then on the right. The nurse tries to point and then move his head in that direction. Thomas pays no heed to the pointing finger and arm suspended just above his face. The nurse gets the toys. The physical therapist tries to position Thomas's arms underneath him to lift his torso toward the rattle. Thomas grits his teeth. He makes no attempt to turn his torso over. She continues the upward push on his torso. Able to push him almost to the apex of the rotation, she eases his body back to the mat. She then moves to the other side, excusing herself in front of the nurse, and places herself in Thomas's line of vision. She tries to tuck his arms underneath him to enable his roll in the direction to which she wants him to turn. She arranges his legs, tucking them underneath his torso. She says to the nurse, "I just figured out what this does. I'm trying to figure things out," as she maneuvers the body into the position for a roll. Without any instruction to Thomas, she moves his legs and arms into the direction of the roll and tries to push him. Thomas does not budge. She says to the nurse, "The cause of the problem is the muscles."

The nurse asks, "Can he get up any further from that position?"

"No," says the physical therapist as she shakes her head. The nurse makes notes on her clipboard. They both get up, staring at Thomas for awhile. They shake their heads. Thomas looks down and away from them.

The physical therapist walks out, but returns awhile later to exercise Thomas's arms and legs by flexing them into the positions that she tried during the examination. She continues extending and flexing arms and legs, one after the other, while Thomas looks away, for twenty minutes.

The nurse comes in and says to Patrick, "How you doing?" and leans down to examine his diaper rash. She tells the attendant not to put him in the wheelchair, but to let him crawl around. Shortly thereafter, while the attendants are still changing residents, the teachers come in to collect residents for the afternoon socialization group. One teacher points out to her aide that Thomas is not changed yet. She states emphatically, "I'm not going to change him," and walks out of the room. She returns ten minutes later.

The physical therapist and the nurse approach Thomas with a greeting but with no explanation about what they are going to do. They seem to assume that no explanation for the intrusion is required. That Thomas rolls away rather than cooperates is a surprise. They decide to take control of the situation by moving into position to hold him down. Thomas rolls away from them three times. Although he has demonstrated his version of the roll three times, they continue to assess his ability to roll in a prescribed way by moving his arms and legs into position, then settle on exercising his arms and legs outside the context of his roll. Thomas allows the therapy but registers his dissatisfaction by turning his head.

The following physical therapy evaluations of his roll are technically correct; but no mention is made of their context.

Evaluation: description of roll

Roll indicated from the supine to the prone and vice versa, but only to right side of the trunk and fixed position of knees prevents him from being able to roll towards the left.

Rolls using the extensor pattern, hyperextending his back and trunk and using strong musculature tone on left side of his trunk to pull him over.

Rolling is very stressful activity for him because of his basic lack of control over his pelvis and lower extremities.

Using his right shoulder muscles to assist, he adducts his right arm to get underneath himself and pushes with his shoulder extensors ... rolls far enough over for gravity to assist the movement, he just flops the rest of the way showing no further control.

Recommendation:

Tolerance for prone position to 1/2 hour; improve upright position in wheelchair; increase ability to mobilize scooter with left arm 10 feet; increase reach with right arm to three times; increase to hold head up and in midline to 30 seconds consistently. (Physical therapy report, 1980)

The roll is evaluated in isolation, divorced from what the resident was doing or how he might use the roll in daily activities. The recommendations are thus based on what is best for Thomas *in therapy*. What is incorporated into the program are the recommendations of the therapist – for example, tolerance of the prone position, increased use of the right arm, and positioning of the head. The program builds on these recommendations. His performance in therapy does not correspond to his demonstrated ability outside of therapy. Often, the mismatch is perpetuated by objectives that never correspond to natural ability even though they may hint at it. One reason is that observation and assessment are only seen within the context of the lesson and the evaluations themselves. Since we have already observed the play event that Thomas chooses to initiate, this ability can be observed.

The play event between Danial and Thomas spans two and a half hours. Motivation and incentive are sustained; the physical exertion is maintained by the two boys to travel great distances, to play, roll over and take turns. Progress notes for June 1978 suggest that Thomas can only mobilize himself a distance of five feet in the typical 20- or 30-minute lesson. In the reports throughout 1979 Thomas is described as requiring physical assistance to pass an object and to maintain his weight on his elbows and his head in midline for one to two minutes. He mobilizes a scooter board two feet in a therapist-directed activity, but in the play event with Danial he travels independently a distance of 30 or more feet.

Evaluation of what the residents are able to do is limited to performance within the activities arranged by teachers and therapists. Recording ability in terms of objectives with criteria for performance in the context of the lesson reveals very little of the ways in which Thomas goes about what he has to do. That Thomas will reach for and hold his favorite toy 100% of the time and that he will maneuver himself to get close to the group are hinted at, but these notations pale in significance when contrasted with the reality. Observation is conducted within the criteria of the lesson. Performance is judged relative to the professionals' criteria of involvement.

Socialization class

This socialization class was conducted right after the teachers' lunch break and the residents' rest period. It was an activity in which all the teachers could combine their separate classes into one group to promote peer interaction among residents. Since each class had a socialization program to teach the same skills, the teachers found it advantageous to combine the activity.

The residents, while living in one of the most public of places with the highest concentration of intervention and involvement in their daily lives, are not presented in the assessment, instruction, reports, or records as individuals living in a social environment. Even the programmed area of "Socialization," designed to teach them peer interaction, does not record their social ability in its complexity. The very acts which demonstrate their ability to interact and identify who they play with are not observed in this setting because of the preconceived format for observation, the categories for behavior observed, and the time, place, and schedule of observations. The reports do not connect what is done by the individual with anyone else.

The school year 1979–80 was the first full year of concentration on socialization of the residents as part of the sensory stimulation curriculum. The socialization program focuses on "the client's social behaviors and skills" in the areas of body awareness, staff interaction, peer interaction, sexuality, interaction with peers of the opposite sex, participation, use of leisure time, and community recreation. The resident is evaluated in terms of demonstrated ability in each area. For each area, a resident achieves one of three skill levels: "no response in the social situation," "follows a moving person," and "regards other people as objects to be explored." When a resident completes the socialization program – that is, when he can play games, initiate behaviors, and play on his own – he moves into a basic skills curriculum.

The teachers enter the ward to pick up the residents for socialization class. Except for Patrick and Julie and Pamela, they are lifted onto their wheelchairs and bed stretchers and wheeled across the hall. Patrick is placed in a wheelchair nonetheless and left to sit (despite the doctor's recommendation moments

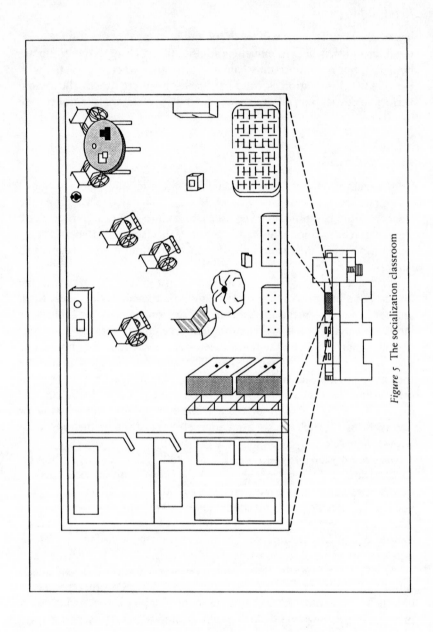

Figure 5 The socialization classroom

before that Patrick not be placed in a wheelchair). After about an hour, the psychologist passes through the activity area, takes him out of the chair, and shakes his head as he lowers him back on to the mat. As she watches the others go out of the apartment and into the hallway, Julie starts to cry. (Julie is over 22 years old, and can no longer participate in the educational programs.) An attendant comes up to her, sits down next to her and wipes her eyes. She looks up at me and says, "She's crying because she can't go to school. There's no program at all for her, so she's just left. Makes you realize something is going on inside." The older woman attendant sits with her for awhile and then gets up to bring her juice and feeds her with a straw.

Pamela lies on the waterbed, shaking her plastic ring of different colored keys, barely able to lift them off the shifting surface of the waterbed. She shakes her head back and forth and emits a slight groaning sound, trying to attract attention of those passing her by. Finally, the grandmother who always feeds her comes in and walks over to her saying, "I see you. I see you. I see you, don't worry, my little brat." "Some people don't like her," she says to me as I watch the transfer of the residents. "I like her and she knows it. All right. Don't worry." She sits down beside her, slides her hands underneath her gently, lifts her into her wheelchair. She takes her for a walk up and down the corridors of the building.

The socialization class across the hall from the apartment was arranged by the teachers for the upcoming activities (see fig. 5). The residents wait in the wheelchairs, motionless. These teachers take them out of their chairs one by one and lift them to mats on the floor, onto the waterbed, or onto cushions in the center of the classroom. Four are left in the wheelchairs and maneuvered around a table in the far corner of the room: Barbara, Dana, Martin, and Wendall. Todd is wheeled next to Deborah, near the table but facing over the mats. Jamie is rolled in around them to the head of the line. Jamie then is separated from Deborah by a few feet, near where the teacher stands overseeing the other residents. The teacher moves Joseph to the center of the room and places him in a rocking chair beside the mat. One teacher on the mat rocks Ryan in her lap. The second lies on the waterbed with Melissa and Maxine. The third teacher, the organizer, to whom all questions and comments are addressed, stands between the wheelchairs of Deborah and Jamie.

Three aides and one student teacher are in the classroom on this particular day. One teacher-aide and the student teacher stand by the table and begin an activity of passing and taking objects. They stand behind and between the wheelchairs around the table and help pass objects, giving constant directions over the shoulders of the residents. The second aide sits on the mats facing opposite the organizing teacher. Danial and Thomas are on either side of him. He assembles a ball and bowling pins around him. The third teacher-aide stands beside Todd and, looking into his face, takes out hand lotion and starts to rub it over his hands and arms, speaking to him in a very quiet voice. She does not take her eyes off him the entire time, but keeps rubbing the lotion into his skin for the next half hour. At one point, she switches to shaving cream. At the end of the half hour, she wipes off his arms with a wet face cloth. Meanwhile, Thomas and Danial spend the entire time on either side of the male teacher-aide

who has collected a ball, the bowling pins, and a telephone to conduct his
interaction with the two of them. Danial's and Thomas's preference for one
another is stated obliquely without mention of names in Danial's annual review
of April 1980–81: "Enjoys socialization with preference to one peer. They both
enjoy the same activities, such as passing a ball to each other and rolling a
bowling ball towards bowling pins."

Thomas and Danial lie looking at the teacher-aide. The teacher-aide reaches
past the bowling balls and pins, telephone and ball for the xylophone and the
mallet. He brings it between both of them saying, "You're going to work
together." He reaches over and pulls each one closer to the other. He also
reaches over and brings out a toy beehive with a bee perched on top of the hive.
Pulling the string from inside the hive makes the wings of the bee on the top fly
up and down. Holding the hive before each boy, he gives them a turn to pull the
string and watch the wings flutter up and down.

The aide then picks up the tamborine and shows them how to hit it. First
Danial hits it, then Thomas. The aide says only, "Hit the tamborine." He gives
Danial the stick to hit the tamborine. Danial reaches for the stick, but instead
picks up a block near him and throws it away in the opposite direction. He
reaches for the stick again but instead of taking it, turns completely over and
away from the aide. Danial reaches for the xylophone behind him and over his
shoulder. The aide tells him to get the xylophone six times before Danial pulls it
close to him. The aide helps him to bring the xylophone to the space in between
the two boys. The aide finally grabs it himself and brings it around as Danial
turns back over. The aide turns to Thomas and tells him, "Give me your hand."
The aide takes the xylophone mallet to place in Thomas's hand. While he turns
to do this, Thomas picks up a block next to him and bangs it on the xylophone.
When the aide tries to give him the mallet, Thomas looks away, but turns back
and hits the xylophone with his hand. At the same time, Danial grabs the mallet
that fell to the ground next to him. The aide puts the mallet in Thomas's other
hand. Thomas allows the aide to move his hand to the board and hits the
instrument as directed by the aide.

After a few hits, the aide moves the xylophone in front of Danial and places
his hand over Danial's to facilitate striking with the mallet on the xylophone,
telling him, "Do this." The teacher who has been watching while rubbing lotion
on Jamie says to the aide. "They're not working together today?" The aide
answers, "No," and shakes his head. "Try the boxes," responds the teacher.
"The boxes will make them work together." "Oh yeah, the boxes," the aide
replies.

The toy selected for play by the teacher is the beehive. The teacher-aide
is the same individual who conducted the classroom lesson in the
morning. He announces what they are going to do, that is, work together.
Each pulls the string in turn. The teacher-aide introduces the tamborine.
After one round of participation, Danial throws a block to register
independent objection. Then he selects the xylophone.

The aide uses hand-over-hand assistance to ensure Thomas's participation. Thomas appears to respond to his insistence by rejecting the mallet and picking up the block. Thomas eventually complies and the aide determines that it is Danial's turn. The two boys' shared patterns of interacting do not correspond to the teacher's methods for conducting the lesson. Simply, the two boys are not working in the ways in which the teacher-aide expects.

Meanwhile, Thomas grabs the tamborine and pulls it toward him. "Stop it," the aide demands. "What do you think you are doing?" Thomas, with the tamborine, moves away from the aide. The aide gets up and collects a set of blocks like the two near the boys. Danial grabs the mallet and goes after the tamborine which Thomas has. The aide returns and reaches them just in time to pull them apart. Thomas tries to hold onto the tamborine and Danial tries to get it away from him. The aide takes the tamborine from Thomas and gives it to Danial, along with a mallet, telling him to hold the stick and hit the tamborine. Danial does that. Watching this, Thomas moves closer. The aide moves them further apart.

The aide takes Danial's hand and rotates it. The aide then lifts up the beehive toy and tells Danial to watch the bee as he pulls the string. He then turns to Thomas and tells him not to hit the string as he holds the beehive up and away from Danial. Danial goes after the string of the beehive while Thomas tries to hit it. The aide moves it further away from Danial. Danial stops, but goes after the blocks by rolling over towards them behind the aide. He turns back over and goes after the block by Thomas. Seeing this, Thomas pulls the few blocks near him closer to him. He reaches and pulls one next to him. Thomas reaches for it again and puts it over his head, then throws it in the direction of Danial. With this, the aide says, "Not to throw, share."

Danial grabs for the box of blocks that the aide has placed in front of him and pulls them toward himself. The aide tells him, "Give it to Thomas." Both Thomas and Danial grab at the same box. Danial stops pulling and goes after a second box. Thomas, watching Danial, stops what he is doing and shakes the first box all the harder. The aide picks up the boxes of blocks and moves them closer to the two boys. Danial starts into a roll to get the tamborine. The aide anticipates this and lifts the tamborine over him and right beside him. Danial picks it up and throws it into the box. The aide turns away from Danial and faces Thomas. The aide gets the tamborine which has been thrown away by Danial and puts it in front of Thomas, puts the mallet in his hand and directs him to hit it by making the hand motions for him.

Behind the aide's back, Danial rolls over closer to the blocks and starts to take them out of the box and throw them. After the third one flies by, the aide turns around and yells, "Hey, stop." The aide picks up Danial and moves him across the mat in the opposite direction from Thomas. On the mat, Danial grabs a play telephone and starts to jingle it by shaking it and pulling it across the mat. The aide returns to Thomas and has him hit the tamborine.

The teacher, who has been watching says, "They're not together today, are they?" "Not really," replies the aide, who once more moves Danial farther away from Thomas and the phone. Danial's phone is now a few feet away from him. Danial looks away from the phone and rolls next to Thomas, facing him. The aide stands and watches.

Rhetorically the aide asks what Thomas is doing. While the aide collects the blocks, Danial grabs the mallet and goes after Thomas's tamborine. The aide immediately separates them. Arbitrarily, the aide gives the tamborine and the mallet to Danial. Danial immediately hits the tamborine with the mallet. Thomas watches and moves to get what Danial has. The aide then pulls them further apart. Thomas does not give up. The aide shows Danial how to rotate his hand on the mallet to hit the tamborine. Then he substitutes the beehive for the tamborine. Thomas gets into the act by hitting the beehive toy, thus interfering with Danial's participation. Danial does more than lose interest; he goes after the blocks near Thomas. Thomas, seeing that Danial is intent on getting the blocks, does not wait for him to come any closer. He picks up a block and throws it at Danial.

Danial goes right after the box of blocks that the aide brings in. The teacher-aide continues to adhere to the purposes and the direction of the lesson. Danial switches the focus and goes after the second box. Thomas shakes the first box of blocks to make Danial aware of what he has. The aide picks up both boxes and places the blocks closer to the two boys. Danial moves beyond the box of blocks to get the tamborine. Rather than letting him go, the aide picks it up and moves it closer to him. He did not anticipate that Danial would throw the tamborine at the box of blocks. The aide takes the tamborine and begins to work with Thomas. Danial picks up blocks and throws them in the direction of Thomas and then the aide. The aide picks up Danial to move him away. On the mat, Danial makes his presence known by jingling the telephone.

Overseeing the lesson, the teacher attends to what Danial and Thomas do while she conducts her own lesson. Her disclaimer that they are not working together today belies what is really going on. What they are doing is not entirely clear, or not as clear as their play on their own, because the aide constantly arranges and rearranges the lesson. When the aide separates the two boys and substitutes toys, he interferes with what they are doing. Even in a directed lesson, Danial and Thomas find opportunities to initiate their own pattern of play. Their interaction recalls their patterned play with the lawn mowers described in chapter 3.

Seeing that they are moving together, the aide says, "Let's try one last fling."
The teacher suggests, "See if they will get the lawn mower. Did you let them play with the lawn mower?" The aide gets the lawn mower and puts it between them. Thomas curls up and appears to pay no attention. Danial picks up the mallet and hits the xylophone. Then he crawls over after the lawn mower, picks it up by the handle and rolls it up and down, back and forth. Danial starts to

roll it in the direction of Thomas. The aide picks up the xylophone. The noise of the lawn mower startles Thomas. He jerks to look up at it as it rolls.

Danial starts to raise it over Thomas's head. The time is 3:25 p.m. The teachers begin to pick up what they are doing and move the residents closer to the door. The socialization group is over for the day. Danial continues rolling the lawn mower over Thomas's head then pulling it away. Thomas moves down on the mat closer to Danial. The attendant comes in to collect Thomas, tells him to wake up since he is now lying still. The attendant looks down at him and says, "Wake up, it's time to go." The attendant goes to get Anna, separating her from Roger. Thomas rolls completely over again in the direction of Danial. Danial rolls the lawn mower towards him and pulls it away. The teacher starts to lift Thomas then stops, realizing she cannot do it alone. She stands over the two boys, waiting for someone to help her. Thomas grabs the lawn mower and Danial pulls it back away from him. They both smile at each other. Thomas rolls over three times, closer to Danial. Danial moves parallel to Thomas. Danial puts the lawn mower over Thomas's head and shakes it. Danial lets it fall and hits Thomas in the chest. Thomas reaches for the lawn mower while looking at Danial. The organizing teacher joins the other teacher standing over them and says, "You guys going to play now? Well, O.K., we'll put you on the mats together." The aide who has been working with them adds, "No, it's over. See you later. It's time to go." The teacher-aide holds the bed stretcher as the two teachers lift Thomas into it and roll him out the door.

Next, Danial is picked up and placed in his bed stretcher and wheeled across the hall. They are placed in opposite corners of the activity area. The lawn mower stays in the classroom.

The socialization group has ended. The teacher decides there was not time today to give them the ice cream. "It was very frozen," reports the teacher-aide.

After all the residents are wheeled into the activity area, Danial picks up Patrick's toy rubber duck and plays with it for the next half hour. He makes the duck squeak and rolls it through his hands and pushes it along in front of him. As I stand bent over the room divider, watching Danial play with the toy duck, the older woman attendant comes up to me and says, "These are all my children." I nod in agreement as she pulls her coat on and walks out the door. The night shift are already preparing the residents for the evening meal.

The aide suggests one more attempt to continue the lesson and the teacher recommends the lawn mower. The aide places the lawn mower between them. At first Thomas does not pay attention. Finally, Danial begins hitting the xylophone with a mallet. He crawls over to the lawn mower and rolls it back and forth beside him. Danial moves the toy closer to Thomas. Clearing up as the end of the lesson approaches, the aide takes the xylophone. Reacting to the noise of the lawn mower, Thomas looks over.

Danial raises the lawn mower over Thomas's head. (Watching the time scheduled for the activity, the teacher also starts to clear things away. Now neither the aide nor the teacher watch Danial and Thomas.) Thomas moves down closer to Danial. An attendant comes in to bring Thomas back to the apartment. He thinks Thomas is asleep because he is now lying still. He goes on to collect Anna. Thomas rolls completely in the direction of Danial. Danial poses the next challenge by pushing the lawn mower and pulling it away from Thomas. The teacher comes over and starts to lift Thomas in the middle of this activity, without even considering that she interrupts the play she has encouraged earlier. Thomas grabs at the lawn mower but Danial pulls it back. They smile at one another.

Thomas rolls three times in rapid succession to get closer to Danial. Danial moves parallel to Thomas. Danial puts the lawn mower over Thomas's head and lets it fall. Thomas reaches for the lawn mower. At this point, the teachers step in to move Thomas. Both boys are picked up and returned to the activity area of the apartment in which they live. Danial plays with a duck. The change of shifts brings a new staff to the apartment.

Even though Danial and Thomas play in their own way in the socialization class designed to teach them to play, the teacher has only noted their lack of cooperation within the context of the lesson. The program is over now. What she misses is a repetition of the patterned play which has been established at least two years (and which was observed in the first phase of the study).

The teacher directs the activity in terms of the objective to play with selected toys in a particular way, for example, pulling the beehive's string, or tapping the xylophone, or tamborine. Danial and Thomas are each far more intent on what the other does and on the ways in which they can get what the other has than on their participation in what the teacher wants. They have already evolved a way of interacting and playing.

The teacher and the aide conclude that they are "not working together today." They are working together but not in the ways in which they are expected to perform. In the course of the event the teacher moves from directing the activity and introducing new objects to follow what they are up to – for example, when Danial moves away from the beehive toy to the xylophone.

Beginning with the blocks, the teacher defines what they are expected to do – not to throw blocks but to share them. The definition of play and sharing in the interaction is developmentally and culturally normative. The solution is to direct the introduction of toys and direct the way they are going to interact. Socialization occurs as individual involvement with the teacher. The residents are asked to participate in activities and to develop skills which are based, not on their evolved or natural ways of making their needs felt in their daily life in the apartment, but on predefined developmental skills. The focus on skills precludes a full interpretation of their natural ability. The teacher is trying not just to get them to do something but to get them to do it in a particular way.

The reports on the lessons illustrate the continued attention to objectives for specific abilities over programmed periods of time. Two years after the play event between Danial and Thomas, the reports on the objectives still do not correlate with what they are actually able to do. The objectives outline the number of sessions, the length of each session, and the criteria, none of which coincides with the performance of Thomas in the play event with Danial in the first period of observation. The lessons are repeated, the criteria get stiffer, and the documentation more elaborate and explicit, addressing more and finer distinctions in skills.

The two boys play in a way which is familiar to them. The cycle of invitation and response is repeated with the tamborine, the string of the beehive, and the blocks. They demonstrate the ability to understand the context of the lesson and what is being asked of them, they are aware of what the other has, they choose to participate in the lesson or not. Within the breaks in the lesson, they seize the opportunity to engage with one another. With the lawn mower they immediately initiate their pattern of play. They attract one another's attention, position themselves to continue the interaction, and challenge each other by moving the lawn mower. They actively engage in circumventing what the teacher does, and maintain their own strategies for interaction. The boys initiate the same pattern of play in the presence of the teachers as they did on their own during rest period. What they do in the lesson reflects what they do on their own. The teacher focuses on their explicit behavior in the context of the lesson, and misses the underlying meaning implicit in how they perform.

The residents have evolved ways of interacting with objects and with each other. The shared and learned nature of Danial's and Thomas's play with the lawn mower is different from the required performance of beating a mallet on the xylophone, pulling the string on the beehive, or playing with the blocks. Their play with the lawn mower contains all the constitutive elements of peer interaction. The sequences reveal complicated interactions involving positioning to play, signaling to exchange, rest from play, prompting to renew the activity, and recovery from interruption.

In lessons which the teachers plan for the residents, the professionals try to involve the residents in activities and lessons which may have no intrinsic connection with the residents' everyday life. The play with the lawn mower implies connection and value, meaning and significance. Danial and Thomas like to play with it. The teachers do not teach them new ways to play with the lawn mower or begin the instruction with demonstration of a new game with the lawn mower, nor is it evident in the records that they have ever observed the full range of the residents' ability with the lawn mower. Thus the activities the teacher presents do not match the ability of the residents or the range and the repertoire of their behavior, nor do these activities take into account the ways in which the residents already perform – ways which show the residents capable of interaction with each other and on their own, in their own way.

By 1980 peer interaction has been developed into a formal program in which residents engage with peers selected for them, within the time constraints of lessons, and around assigned criteria for success determined by professionals. The social context of the classroom and the demands for interaction and performance do not consider the unique qualities of the interaction because of the superimposition of labels and descriptions of handicap. Professional intervention does not incorporate provision for social interaction, nor does it consider the context of an event, or the quality of the professionals' participation in the residents' lives.

The list of need areas for the residents grew in parallel with the increase in professional staff whose responsibility it was to identify the need areas. The identified need areas fluctuated in the course of the study, depending on residents' needs, program schedules, and the availability of the professionals to conduct the lessons. The rise of professional status within the building and the identification of a program with a discipline limited the focus of each of the professionals to tasks, programs, and activities within his or her area.

Summary

From 1978 to 1983 the social organization of the institution evolved as a program for the residents, based on the concepts of deinstitutionalization, mainstreaming, and normalization, with an underlying principle of individualization. On the basis of a clinical determination of functional ability, an individualized educational program is designed for each resident. The interdisciplinary process of diagnosis and assessment, the development of objectives to teach specific skills, the annual review, and continuous evaluation define the social process, the role and relationship of staff to resident. Interactions are short, focused, and part of a general routine for the conduct of an examination or therapy. It involves the staff in a prescribed routine with the residents, but also with the other members of the examination team. The behaviors are reported as isolated facts concerning the individual. They are judged by the dichotomous criteria – "do or not do" – criteria not suited to the levels of their complexities nor representing residents' patterns in the context of their daily life. The structuring of the residents' daily schedule becomes

Summary

increasingly defined formally around the conduct of educational and therapeutic activities with professionals.

The formal structure of the institution is built upon an understanding of what the residents *do* in the context of programmed activities. The focus is on the handicap rather than on the individual. The residents are still evaluated in terms of a bifurcated system of normal and abnormal. While attention is shifted to the individual's needs in a specific program, such "individualization" is not based upon a full awareness of the individual.

The social organization of the institution and the principles on which it is based function to ameliorate handicaps, to minimize diversity, to attend to individual differences by systematically structuring an approach to that diversity. The result is a fusion of formal and informal methods of care and treatment into a continuous, systematic orientation toward the individual. The increased formalization of the social organization of the institution places a premium on maintenance of the apartment in conformity with administrative expectations, and on interpretations of the requirements of the law to provide individual care and treatment.

Often the residents experience the institutional organization, programs, and schedule as an interruption to their own activities. In some cases it results in tension, in others, outright resistance, and in others, manipulation and calculation; but it exists as an increasing influence in the social interaction with the residents throughout the implementation of the programs. In these interactions with the residents, institutional social organization and processes meet their greatest challenge.

5

Summary: inquiry, knowledge, and practice

The historical context

Howe believed the imperfect combination of human systems, which resulted from the organic nature of idiocy, made the ensuing manifestation of functional ability limitless. The severely and profoundly mentally retarded and multiply handicapped in this study represent a limitless combination of differences and involvements. Structuring an approach to their diversity is found in the evolution of practice based on clinical observation and interpretation of their behavior and ability.

Pinel's clinical distinction of mental functioning found fruition in the testing of intelligence and the standardization of assessment of mental abilities. Today the application of standardized measures of intelligence to the severely and profoundly mentally retarded and multiply handicapped results in the conclusion that the individual is "untestable." Test failure leads to the proliferation of skills checklists, developmental assessment scales, and matrices of adaptive behavior and functional ability. While profiles of functional ability serve as a reference point for the determination of practice, the diversity and variation within an individual's performance *challenge* the assumption that clinical comparisons represent all that he or she is able to do.

Itard based his educational program for Victor on clinical observation and interpretation of his student's functional ability. He planned educational tasks, developed a sequence of instruction, and managed his interaction with Victor. Itard's goal was to assimilate Victor into appropriate social and cultural patterns of behavior.

Today, individualized educational programs reflect increased sophistication and formalization of Itard's clinical and scientific method applied to education. Similarly, goals and objectives within the individualized educational program represent a sequence of skills and abilities, designated tasks, and strategies for interaction, designed to enhance normal functioning.

Séguin sharpened the focus on functional ability through clinical analysis. His efforts to develop educational material and methods were aimed at freeing the mind and the potential of the individual from the limitations and constraints of the defect. On the basis of the relationship of functional behavior to specific organs, Séguin designed an instructional approach to train the organ. Today, the aim of instructional strategies and methods is to affect underlying pathology through enhancement of functional ability. Assessment of behavior and ability in this way is judged as practical, and advantageous to the individual, by the professional staff.

The attention to the total individual which was advocated by Montessori to accommodate differences is reflected in the interdisciplinary and multi-disciplinary assessments and educational planning for the severely and profoundly mentally retarded and multiply handicapped. Indeed, today, every aspect of ability and functioning is scrutinized intensely within this setting to find a way to develop potential. Given the context of the interaction and the focus of the observation during assessment, the severely and profoundly mentally retarded and multiply handicapped – the extreme of variation and difference – repeatedly fail to demonstrate the full range of their ability under this intense scrutiny. The clinical picture which evolves in the case study of the individual represents only one form of interpretation of who they are and what they do.

Howe's categorization of the facts of idiocy did not deter him from consideration of the independent character of the will, the natural signs and expressions representative of a different form of language. Again and again, the form and the content of interaction and participation with one another represent individual will and volition. Form in their expression and patterns in their interaction which have evolved over time should be the basis for determining the nature of interaction and participation with others in any setting.

The underlying principle of education advocated by Fernald was habit training. For Fernald, the absence or loss of ability represented deficit and deficiency. Today, habit training is reflected in the repetition of practice of isolated skills and tasks, and in routines for the consistent management of interaction and communication within a prescribed framework. Structuring the approach to diversity through habitual forms of communication, interaction, and participation is an accepted standard of practice, and is viewed as a means to achieve consistency.

The consistency in our approach to their multiple involvements – that is, their organic handicaps and resulting forms of expressions – lies in clinical observation and analysis of behavior. The history of special education is the continual refinement of observation, explanation, and development of abilities and behaviors in this clinical context.

The singularity of this clinical perspective and the continual application of mainstream cultural standards to the interpretation of residents' experience, the management of their behavior, and the direction of educational and therapeutic practice, run the risk of misrepresenting and misinterpreting their experience. Consequently, at the level of interaction and participation, we miss the essential nature of their differences.

The study of the severely and profoundly mentally retarded population has traditionally been conducted in clinical, quantitative, and experimental modes (Mann and Sabatino, 1973). In a 1977 review of 500 empirical studies of the severely and profoundly mentally retarded, conducted between 1955 and 1974, Berkson and Landesman-Dwyer found that most description and assessment were based on formal testing of behavior in four areas: the correspondence between medical syndromes and behavior, the level of functioning in sensory and perceptual areas, the measure of intelligence on standardized tests, and ratings of adaptive behaviors. A fifth area was a search for environmental factors that evoked and maintained a behavioral response. Behavior was understood in terms of the prescribed labels and definitions of medical, psychological, and educational categories and norms.

Since the time of Itard, researchers and practitioners have been absorbed in an approach which has almost closed the door on any alternative forms of inquiry. Berkson and Landesman-Dwyer confirmed that the accepted standard for care continues to be custodial and medical. In contrast to clinical experimental designs, for instance, only three studies in this review employed direct, naturalistic observation of behavior (Landesman-Dwyer, 1974; MacAndrew and Edgerton, 1964; Wills, 1973).

Other research methods commonly used for studying the mentally retarded include standardized psychometric instruments, task performance tests, questionnaires, interviews, adaptive behavior measures, and clinical judgements (Sackett, 1978a, 1978b). The appropriateness of these measures with the severely and profoundly mentally retarded was questioned by Sackett because they do not adequately capture or accurately predict the full range of actual behavioral adaptation to real life situations. Except for adaptive behavior measures, all of these methods depend heavily on verbal competence. Although direct observation using quantitative methods is advocated by Berkson (1978:403–409) as a means of inquiry beyond formal testing, observation relies on labels and definitions from the "normal" mainstream culture. Knowledge gained in this manner unwittingly interprets the behavior of the severely and profoundly mentally retarded in the researcher's own cultural terms, categories, and meanings. The dominance of the clinical orientation has led to a singularity of perspective on this population, even as new requirements for care and education are mandated.

Landesman-Dwyer (1974) made one of the first major attempts to study the institutionalized, nonambulatory, multiply handicapped as one "biobehavioral" category of profound mental retardation. In this study, the behavior of a resident in a play-pen, alone or with toys, is rated on standardized measures and compared with the behavior of normal individuals. Landesman-Dwyer concluded that individuals show marked increase in attention to and interest in external stimuli, such as the placement of toys. Landesman-Dwyer recognized the inappropriateness of the test and rating measures with this population. She recognized the necessity to gain a full understanding of the behavioral repertoire, but relied on measures which did not lend themselves to this goal.

Subsequent researchers chose to identify increasingly smaller facets and domains of the individual in experimental and quantitative studies. Qualitative methods, in the tradition of Edgerton, have been applied to the socio-behavioral study of the mentally retarded. These studies focus attention on the unique life circumstances of the mildly and the moderately mentally retarded. In these studies, conversations and dialogue are the data by which the researcher understands their view of their own work, sexuality, and life circumstances.

Research analysis of communication, social competence, and interaction in the classroom and learning environments found its application to the mentally retarded population. The characteristics and features of communication were reexamined (Cole and Traupman, 1980; Longhurst, 1974; Macmillan, 1977; Rueda 1982, Rueda and Chan, 1980). These studies focus on the social and interactive meaning expressed by the borderline, educable, and trainable mentally retarded. The primary subject of the research has been social competence, adaptive behavior, and vocational, occupational, and interpersonal adjustment (Greenspan, 1979; Simeonson, 1979), and the social context of classroom interaction (Cole and Traupman, 1980; Levine and Langness, 1983: Longhurst, 1972, 1974; Price-Williams and Sabsay, 1979; Rueda and Chan, 1980; Rueda, 1982). The severely and profoundly mentally retarded and multiply handicapped have received little attention. The limitations of comparison with others were found in the investigation of nine Down's Syndrome individuals by Price-Williams and Sabsay (1979).

Unraveling the complexity of the communication strategies of the severely and profoundly mentally retarded and multiply handicapped requires attention to the differential effect of their disability. The study of the residents of institutions, specifically the mentally retarded, only lightly touches the identification of their repertoire of communication.

In the preceding discussion we have suggested that in this linguistically impaired population there is a great deal of communication, both verbal and nonverbal, and that this communication is a great deal more complex than previous clinical studies on the language of the mentally retarded would suggest. This communication, moreover, is subject to the same requirements and follows some of the same basic patterns as that of normally competent adults and children. The communicative strategies used by these individuals tend to be more like those used by young children just acquiring language. The use of these strategies, however, may be occasioned less by communicative or cognitive incompetence than by the communicative distress arising from the retardates' linguistic impairment.

Although these individuals are often described as having the mental age of a child of 2 or 3 years, they are not children. They have many years of interacting with the environment and with other individuals (although in some ways their experience may be actually more limited than that of a child). In addition, although we are not prepared to identify the differences, it seems that their conversation is different from that of children in some ways. In some ways it seems more "sophisticated," in others more simple or disordered. One cannot discount, for example, the effects of such cognitive disabilities as short term memory impairment.

Researchers in the field of language and mental retardation have been concerned primarily with the relationship between cognitive impairment and linguistic deficits, and with developing language intervention programs. They have focused on the language and speech of individuals in isolation. Procedures for evaluating language behavior have shown little regard for the situated use of language, and for the communicative abilities underlying its use. This approach has fostered an image of the retardate as a linguistic incompetent who must be taught the rudiments of language if he is to function in a workshop or in the community. In fact, some retardates may successfully manage verbally mediated social inter-actions with certain environmental and situational requirements. This communi-cative competence is as much a fact to be described and accounted for as their linguistic incompetence. (Price-Williams and Sabsay, 1979:57–58)

Educational literature has focused on the ward and institutional life and has described resident behavior and stereotypical patterns (Davis *et al.*, 1969; Izutsu, 1971; Kaufman and Levitt, 1965), the change under experimental conditions when alternative activities were presented (Hollis, 1976), the establishment of territoriality and aggressive ten-dencies (Rago, 1976, 1977a, 1977b), and the observation of preferences of the multiply handicapped and the deaf-blind (Goode and Gaddy, 1976). These studies focus on very specific behaviors but fail to integrate them into a theory of the relations between competing normal and abnormal systems.

Other studies related to environmental changes and their effect on the residents (Gorton and Hollis, 1965; Levy and McLeod, 1977; National Institute on Mental Retardation, 1978; O'Brien and Poole, n.d.; Tizard and Tizard, 1974), with one study looking at the response of the bed-ridden to their environment (Cleland and Sluyter, 1973). Rogers and Baer (1976) focus on interactions on the ward. The study points to an increase in material resources and staff numbers as significant factors in the decrease of inappropriate behaviors of 28 severely and profoundly mentally retarded (chronological ages 6 to 14). In two of the studies, the residents' perspective was considered. The observation scales (Goode and Gaddy, 1976; Rago, 1977a, 1977b) are in part developed from a consideration of what the residents were actually doing, although the resulting definition and concepts are based on mainstream cultural criteria. One study interviews severely mentally retarded people about their rights to have their perspective considered (O'Donnell, 1976). Others studied the territorial mobility, communication, and involvement in activities as distinguishing features of the humanness of persons with mental retardation.

These studies attempt to underscore the congruence between our intervention and what the residents do. Other studies include attention to the modification of behavior; staff development; achievement on test items; the success of teaching programs, treatments, training devices, and materials; attainment of abilities in activities of daily living, socialization, basic skills and adaptive behavior (Estes, 1970; Fuller, 1949; Killian, 1967; Lederman, 1969; Piper and MacKinnon, 1969; Rice, 1968; Rice and McDaniel, 1966; Rice *et al.*, 1967; Thompson and Grabowski, 1977); the design and arrangement of the environment; and medication and administration of specific drugs. Although the research covers a wide range of important topics, it lacks integration of the diverse findings. The interpretation of the results is in terms of the broader categories of achievement and domains of ability, such as socialization, communication, or social interaction.

Phenomenological analysis of social interaction of the severely retarded in context is found in the work of Goode (1980a) with a similar application to the multiply handicapped deaf-blind (Curtis, 1975 a,b; Goode, 1974, 1975 a,b). Goode documents intersubjective meanings of the individual through social contact and interaction, based on a study of the handicapped individual and the family. Goode relies on personal participation by the researcher to experience and sense the meaning conveyed by the individual from inside the walls of their handicap.

Investigating interactions of two severely disabled non-oral cerebral palsy children, Edelsky and Rosegrant (1980) reported: (1) lack of systematic observation of the children's natural circumstances and communicative ability; (2) use of labels and direction from others, interactions controlled by others, and lack of exposure to normal speech; (3) problems in communication, involving adult perceptions of handicaps and notions about expected relations of children to their world and others; (4) interactions initiated and terminated by others, reflecting assumptions that the individuals lacked volition and will, and that their signal lacked specific meaning and age appropriateness.

Edelsky found that the two children perceived variation in context and differences in interactions; signaled less when not responded to in an interaction; initiated contact to make a request; and were excluded by speakers from the conversations. Interactions reinforced their lack of ability when they did not respond with normal interactive patterns. Edelsky recommended "accommodation" to the multiply handicapped in normal interactions.

Our knowledge of the handicapped as persons is primarily based on two forms of interpretation of their experience: (1) medical – that is, the classification of the handicapping condition; and (2) psychological and educational statements about the characteristics of the condition. Both interpretations rest on models, concepts, and assumptions about appropriate methods of inquiry and the individuals under investigation. Medical understanding interprets the organic cause of the condition in order to classify symptoms. Psychological and educational understanding proceeds from a similar premise – to understand the mental and social characteristics as states, stages, and skills which form the basis for intervention.

The problem is that the labels and categories for their experience – that is, our interpretation of what they do – are grounded not in their experience but in mainstream terms and categories. The terms, categories, and labels can cloud our understanding and perpetuate discussion at a level above what they actually do. The labels which we apply to their experience point to a fundamental flaw in our knowledge, inquiry, and practice.

The residents in transition

On my last visit to apartment M and N in April 1978, I walked into the activity area where I had observed over the course of months. I was sad to leave. In the middle of the floor, Thomas swung the lawn mower up and down but without his pleased smile and contented aspect. I realized I did not hear the popping plastic balls and accompanying melody. The wheel of the lawn mower had fallen off. Thomas tried moving the lawn mower in different directions. Staff passed by but focused their attention on the end-of-the-day activities. Thomas stared into the activity area. Gradually, he stopped moving and lay there in silence until supper was ready. His favorite toy was broken; would it be replaced?

The move of all the residents, anticipated since my arrival in January 1978, occurred early in December 1981. Delays in finding space and alternative programs, funding, and construction plans themselves all postponed the actual departure date. Then, one weekend, the residents were relocated. One setting was additional space at the mental hospital near the school; the other was the floor of the hospital building on the grounds of the institution. One week after the move, I looked down from the administration building into the shell of a building. The cranes were already in place to assist in the demolition. The building would be renovated to planned specifications: subdivided into smaller self-contained units, each with their own dining area, living space and private bedrooms similar to those already on the grounds. What would replace the crowded activity area?

During my review of the archive records, I visited the hospital wing where some of the residents now lived (February 1982). The doors and the halls, grated in wire mesh and locked, kept the residents from the stairways. The highly polished floors reflected my image. The nurse in the attendant station recognized me and said, "Oh, hi. How's the story going?"

I asked if I could see the residents.

"Oh sure. They are just down the hall. They're much better off here than they were in that other place. Did you see it? It was destroyed. Go in and see everyone. It's o.k."

In the activity area of one wing between two sleeping areas were the residents, all lined up and sitting in their newly adapted wheelchairs. I did not recognize any of them. Each wore his or her own personal clothing. Each was strapped into a wheelchair and supported by adaptations to the wheelchairs with extra ties and cushions. Their limbs were strapped to various devices, boards and braces – cushioned headboards, body supports, and plastic braces molded to their contours. The residents tilted over the arms of the chair or leaned in various directions under the pull of the brace. They all had bibs and sheets draped around them. All that was visible were their hands and faces. They sat motionless within the confines of the adaptive equipment.

The attendant entered in sharply pressed white hospital pants and a white shirt. "How do you like it? Sure is different from that other place. Here we take care of the residents. They all have new wheelchairs. They've got new braces. We really got them all cleaned and shaped up. We are really able to do more for them; we got everything they need."

I answered, "It sure is different." He and two other attendants propped up the residents and lined them up for lunch and then pushed them out of the activity area to the other wing. The high headboards on the back of the chairs held their heads straight. In the line, each resident looked at the back of the chair in front.

The nurse came from the attendant station and asked, "Well, how's your story going? Those were hard times. We really didn't have the services and the support to get what we needed for the residents. Now we do. We're really able to care for them now."

Total programming overstepped the bounds of the social and cultural dimensions of the residents' lives. There were no grunts, no groans, the murmur in the apartment was gone. The residents sat in silence. If they slipped out of position, the attendant righted them.

In April 1982, I requested a tour of the institution from the Office of Public Relations, almost five years since my initial tour of the buildings I was to study. I observed the buildings, the workshop, "sensory stimulation to basic skills" classes, and program centers. The supervisor and program coordinators talked in terms of "individualized programs for the residents" or the "program of behavior management." All of the residents in the institution were programmed.

The delivery of service was uniform, the objectives consistently applied, the underlying principles of individualization and the goals of normalization and rehabilitation adhered to. The service and the support required for the appropriate care of the residents was the acquisition of adaptive equipment. Care became the implementation of programs which maintained the residents within therapeutic positions and in approximations of normality. Staff believed this was better. However, the residents were not able to move under the weight of the adaptive devices and the restraints used to maintain their position. They lived within the restrictions of the devices as well as within the limitations of the handicap, and of the rules and programs of the institution.

The real implication for the institution lies in the fact that the goals, the objectives, the mandates, and the delivery of service are deceptive. The illusion is that we have found the starting place for implementation of programs and services in the clinical, psycho-physiological basis of mental retardation. The same gaps in our knowledge exist whether the resident lives in the institution or in a community group home. The lack of basic knowledge of what the residents do ultimately leads to implementation of programs that isolate the residents from one another. The implementation of professional practice is uninfluenced by consideration of its meaning for the individual.

In this setting, what has become special about special education practice is its specialization: close attention to isolated skills and abilities and segments of behavior across the human systems. The severely and profoundly mentally retarded and multiply handicapped, who cannot speak for themselves, are provided services and programs which do not adequately match the reality of their experiences and understanding of the world. The congruence which should exist between programs and services and individual needs becomes circumstantial and ephemeral.

Lacking fundamental understanding grounded in their conduct of daily life, discussion of the severely and profoundly mentally retarded and multiply handicapped is reduced to a concentration on the handicapping condition and the organization and functional aspects of the institution's delivery of services. This fundamental discrepancy in the delivery of service is the result of misunderstanding and misinterpretation of the full range of the resident's ability and performance. The organization for the delivery of service formalizes and objectifies our interpretation of what residents do. Specialization of programs ultimately leads to a new form of isolation and segregation for the residents – restricted not by placement in the institution, but by the nature of professional practice.

A consequence of the use of clinical interpretation of the behavior of the severely and profoundly mentally retarded and multiply handicapped is that fundamental conceptualizations are not changed; no reorientation in understanding is achieved. The distinctions that set them apart proliferate and are perpetuated because of lack of new knowledge upon which to base practice. Mainstream cultural criteria are artificial, and their continual application confuses and glosses over the significance and meaning of their differences.

At the annual review of the residents' educational program, the interdisciplinary team tries to build a picture of the individual from successive lists of skills and abilities. The resulting list is a profile of functional areas but not of the individual. This fragmentation is perpetuated in the process of intervention and the conduct of the program. Since the mode of observation and interpretation of ability does not change, the understanding of the residents is not broadened through practice. The integration of the skills and behaviors in each functional area does not capture the underlying unity in their performance or in the relationships in their human systems. Once established, the separation is maintained in practice.

Getting Danial and Thomas to perform on the lesson does not incorporate what they already bring to the situation – their pattern of play together. They learn the sequence of interaction with the teacher in the same way in which they come to understand each other. Danial and Thomas create in the context of their play and do the same in their interaction with the teacher. To understand their interaction with us is to maintain perspective on our own involvement in the contexts they create and in which we participate.

Misinterpretation of what they do in the lesson ensures misunderstanding of their capabilities and potential. The fact that Danial and Thomas do not play in the prescribed manner within the lesson is reflected in their not meeting the criteria for the objective. Unless the implicit patterns in their behavior are the initial reference point for the description, the asymmetry in interpreting what the residents do is perpetuated in the lesson and formal records of their behavior. An integrated interpretation requires observation of residents on their own, and understanding of the patterns of their interaction with others.

These are individuals who have unique patterns of behavior requiring broader understanding of their forms of communication. Variation in their communication and interaction is natural given the nature of their differences. We must acknowledge that our cultural standards can be applied inappropriately if our interpretations miss the meaning in what they do. In their own way, Danial and Thomas share with each other. To accomplish this play they must understand and interpret each other's ability and the circumstances and the situation each other faces, and communicate implicitly in the meaning of their play. They not only intend to play but share meaning in their play.

Today the concepts of normalization, mainstreaming, and deinstitutionalization are the social principles underlying the nature of services and programs for the residents. Normalization, deinstitutionalization, and mainstreaming for the individual have less to do with placement within or outside of a living, learning, and working environment and more to do with aligning our understanding of their interaction and participation with one another and others.

"Normal" for Danial and Thomas is their shared learned patterns of interaction with each other, within the constraints of their multiple involvements. The definition of normality lies in the implicit meaning in their interaction with one another. Thus, what they do and when they do it should become the basis for any consideration for further normalization of their experience.

The shared learned patterns in their expressions and communications, despite the constraints and influence of pathology, shape their unique patterns of interaction and participation. It is our ability to interpret these patterns that will determine the success of practice. The fulfillment of their potential depends on our understanding their experience. For Danial and Thomas the concept of potential means the opportunity to play and to develop their experience at play. Understanding how to play with Danial and Thomas is the first step in enhancing their play. Interpretations grounded in the context of their own interaction can expand our concept of their normality rather than highlight the essential nature of their differences.

Deinstitutionalization refers to changes in setting and redesign of existing institutional settings to reflect a less restrictive environment for the residents. What is least restrictive to Danial and Thomas has less to do with setting and more to do with the definition and understanding of what they do in the present environment. Understanding the nature of their play, and how to develop and enhance their opportunity for play, is a way to deinstitutionalize their experience.

Any setting can institutionalize experience through the nature of staff interaction and participation. Deinstitutionalization of practice is the removal of restrictions on their participation with one another. Connecting their present experience with new experiences within other environments is the vehicle for development of skills. The success of our participation in the mainstream of their life experience will determine the extent to which participation in other cultural settings will benefit them. To expand their participation we must understand their interaction and participation in the mainstream of apartment life.

Deinstitutionalization comes to mean relinquishing concepts, terms, and categories which have become generalizations about their experience. The assumption that the residents "do not do anything" because they are "really bad off" leads to the belief that "there is nothing going on in the apartment." Consequently, staff must teach them to do everything.

What maintains institutionalization for Danial and Thomas is the formal structure of assessment of skills and abilities and behaviors which translates their experience into less than what it is. The application of the classic definition of the clinical characteristics of their condition limits our understanding. Change in setting may not look deeply enough into the nature of practice. For example, the change in the setting observed in 1979–80 dramatically changed the ability of the residents to interact and participate with one another, and ensured their dependence on staff. Interaction came to mean greater interaction with staff trying to elicit culturally appropriate skills and behaviors within structured contexts. Ironically, these methods were used to teach them to play and interact with one another. In contrast, deinstitutionalization must address the forms of our interaction and participation.

To date, our interaction achieves consistency but may not represent continuity with respect to their experience. Consistency in approach, directed by the individualized educational program, is the trademark of professional practice. Instead, continuity between educational and therapeutic lessons and Danial's and Thomas's experience must guide professional involvement and participation with the residents.

One consistent feature in this intense and professionally dense environment is the singularity of approach to understanding a highly variable and heterogeneous population. Nevertheless, the standardization of practice within the structure and organization of the institution represents a cultural dissonance between the formal structure created to meet the needs of the residents and the ways in which the residents function to meet their needs on their own. Their performance with teachers in lessons and in therapy never matches their ability demonstrated in what they do on their own. The contours which describe how pathology affects functioning give definition to their performance. In this way, they are no longer defined solely by the clinical condition nor by the level of functioning which brings them to this setting and places them in the apartment, but by the form of their participation.

Currently, mainstreaming supports the notion of integration of individuals with developmental disabilities into the mainstream of living, learning, and working environments. Primarily, mainstreaming implies a program which reverses isolation of individuals with developmental disabilities in separate or segregated environments. Participation "in the mainstream" provides the opportunity for the development of ability with peers.

Mainstreaming is a culturally defined concept applied to their experience – communication, interaction, and participation. Mainstreaming depends not only on their ability to participate fully within their present environment but also relates directly to the degree to which others understand the nature of their participation. Mainstreaming cannot be participation in other environments won at the cost of their interaction and participation with one another.

The appropriateness of an environment is determined by the continuity it lends to their experience and by the ways it extends their present communication and interaction. The criteria of appropriateness is less the comparison to others of a similar age, grade, or stage of development, and more the consideration of the range of functioning of the individual given full consideration of their circumstances. Appropriate must mean appropriate for the individual.

The essence of special education practice is interpretation. What staff interpret about what the individual does determines their involvement. The goal of professional involvement must be the encouragement of their ability through programs reflecting their experiences rather than consistency across clinically derived goals and objectives for intervention, education, and management of behavior.

The significant feature of the residents in this setting was not the handicapping condition but what the residents did *despite* the perceived limitations imposed by the handicapping condition. Striking was the degree to which our methods did not capture the uniqueness of their demonstrated ability. Remarkable was the fact that the residents demonstrated their ability repeatedly in the face of our continued adherence to our structured programs and approach to interaction.

In this study, I elucidate a fundamental coherence within the performance of the severely and profoundly mentally retarded and multiply handicapped. This coherence emerges as a pattern of individual behavior formed from experience with others. The evolution of the pattern is in part the result of a particular constellation of clinical characteristics. However, there are other essential human attributes which influence development. Clinical characteristics cannot define other human qualities nor interpret their relative significance for the individual.

Focus on implicit meaning is a new reference point for determining our involvement with their experience. The focus becomes contextually based observation and interpretation of meaning that reveals more than their essential differences. While differences are the profound essence of their humanity, their performance in interactions reveals relationships in the same human systems we share. It demonstrates what we have in common, namely, the desire to participate with others. We can know what they do if we recognize the universals in our common experience beyond the disability.

Significant in this setting is the quality of the interaction of the residents with others. Living in this environment is not a neutral event. What they do is not defined solely in terms of the stereotypes of their labels and the setting. This shorthand for describing what is going on with the residents is precisely the fundamental discrepancy between who the residents are and what they do. Reduction of their experience leads to a fragmented understanding and generalizations; essential unity within their human experience is lost. Lacking alternatives, the conduct of practice splits into the formal representation of the residents in the records based on what is understood in context of professional practice and informal knowledge gained from momentary or chance encounters outside the professional role.

This separation is symbolized in the transition at the institution. Implementation of individualized educational programs limited the residents' interaction to interaction with the staff in the context of teaching a specific skill or offering program options. Even the teaching of play within the socialization group for Danial and Thomas restricts their play. This is significant for each resident because ability grouping is the basis for the resident's placement within programs and determines his or her advancement within the institution. From the residents' perspective, staff interpretation of what they do is the single most important determinant of their quality of life.

To discover the meaning and significance of what they do is a vehicle for understanding their motivations and desires as the basis of our intervention. It acknowledges their participation in the interaction and considers them actors with involvement in their own learning. Danial and Thomas choose whether or not to participate with the teacher-aide in the context of the socialization lesson. In the choice, they demonstrate their knowledge of our socialization process.

It is not how Danial and Thomas play that is similar to all other residents. Rather, it is the attempts by each resident to participate with others which is common to all humanity. Another factor that unites them culturally to the rest of humanity is the evolution of a pattern in their interaction within a particular space and time. A shift in the spatial and temporal dimensions associated with their interactions lifts the focus of attention from characteristics of their pathology that define their differences and places it within the context of interaction.

Conclusion

From the time of Itard, we have attempted to systematically define their differences and acculturate them to our experience. Recognition of their experience challenges us to consider acceptance of it and to fundamentally change the nature of our practice. Professional intervention must move to the level of personal understanding of the implications of policies and procedures for the individual residents if we are to improve the quality of their lives.

I began this study to discover what the residents of this institution do. I was challenged to understand their disabilities in a different way. Interpretation of the ways in which their actions were familiar and recognizable evolved from understanding the context in which their behavior occurred. Gradually, behaviors were distinguished from one another. Those that were meaningful communicated a message with a specific intent and were distinct from those that did not.

Individuals are unique in the ways they express their message. The content is related directly to the fulfilment of their needs, wants and desires. Misunderstanding of the intent and the meaning of the resident by the staff was the basis of the tension in the interaction and misinterpretation of their ability. The misinterpretation is perpetuated within the system for recording the resident's ability.

The opportunity for staff to understand what the residents do on their own as the basis for determining their involvement faded with each passing year of the study. In the end, what the residents did was defined in terms of what the staff did with them. If we continue to define their human experience in terms of the quality of intervention to teach them skills and abilities and to manage behavior, we run the risk of delimiting other essential qualities which contribute to their uniqueness. Danial and Thomas may not lose their pattern of play for now. Rather, the challenge is to ensure its continuance and development within a system that does not acknowledge its significance except as an interference.

The measure of the potential of the severely and profoundly mentally retarded and multiply handicapped rests on the determination of what they can do. It is not the comprehensive listing of skills that determines their ability, but what they do within the constraints of their ability that determines their potential and should guide our intervention. Potential is a concept relative to the full human capacity of the individual to participate – not on someone else's terms – but on their own terms. This is no less true for the severely and profoundly mentally retarded and multiply handicapped than it is for others. Multiple disabilities influence the range of the potential but not its essential quality. Potential cannot be determined relative to a specific set of skills but by the comprehensive consideration of what the person can do in the present.

The severely and profoundly mentally retarded and multiply handicapped are individuals who, if defined in terms of the characteristics of their condition, come to fulfill our expectations and assumptions about them. This definition of them supports our notion of programs and services and the nature of our intervention. With this framework for understanding, it is easy to justify practice, from the vantage point of our experience. Their differences are profound but to focus on these is to miss essential unities and connections to human experience in which they participate. The advancement of practice in special education appears to rest with a reexamination of the state of our knowledge, our methods of inquiry, and the nature of our involvement and participation in their lives.

We must move beyond the first stage of understanding, the clinical description of their condition, in which we have been immersed since the 1800s. Basic knowledge of what they do must be the basis of our inquiry. The advancement of special education practice rests on the degree to which what we do considers what they are already doing.

Bibliography

Anderson, Camilla M. 1963. *Jan, My Brain Damaged Daughter*. Portland: Durham.

Bancroft, Margaret. 1915. *Collected Papers of Margaret Bancroft on Mental Subnormality and the Care and Training of the Mentally Retarded Subnormal Children*. Philadelphia: Ware.

Bateson, Gregory. 1972. *Steps to An Ecology of the Mind*. New York: Ballantine.

1980. *Mind and Nature*. New York: Bantam.

Bateson, Gregory, ed. *Perceval's Narrative*. New York: Morrow.

Bercovici, Sylvia. 1978. *The Deinstitutionalization of Mentally Retarded Persons: Ethnographic Research In Community Environments*. L. L. Langness, ed. Los Angeles: University of California.

Berkson, Gershon. 1978. Social ecology and ethnology of mental retardation. In Gene Sackett, ed., *Observing Behavior*, vol. 1. Baltimore: University Park Press.

Berkson, Gershon and Sharon Landesman-Dwyer. 1977. Behavioral research on severe and profound mental retardation. *American Journal of Mental Deficiency*, 81:428–454.

Biklen, Douglas. 1973. Patterns of Power. Unpublished Ph.D. dissertation, Syracuse University.

Binet, Alfred and T. H. Simon. 1916. *The Development of Intelligence in Children*. Baltimore: Williams and Wilkins.

1916. *The Intelligence of the Feebleminded*. Baltimore: Williams and Wilkins.

Blatt, Burton. 1970. *Exodus from Pandemonium*. Boston: Allyn and Bacon.

1973. *Souls in Extremis*. Boston: Allyn and Bacon.

Blatt, Burton and Fred Kaplan. 1974. *Christmas in Purgatory*. Syracuse: Human Policy.

Blindert, H. Deiter. 1975. Interactions between residents and staff: a qualitative investigation of an institutional setting for retarded children. *Mental Retardation*, 13:38–40.

Bogdan, Robert and Douglas Biklen. 1977. Handicapism. *Social Policy*, 7:14–19.

Bogdan, Robert and Steven J. Taylor. 1975. *Introduction to Qualitative Research Methods*. New York: Wiley.

1982. *Inside Out*. Buffalo: University of Toronto Press.

Bogdan, Robert *et al.* 1974. Let them eat programs: attendants' perspectives and programming on wards in state schools. *Journal of Health and Social Behavior*, 15:142–151.

et al. 1982. The disabled: media's monster. *Social Policy*, 13:32–35.

Boyd, William. 1914. *From Locke to Montessori*. New York: Holt.

Brenneis, Donald. 1982. *Making Sense of Settings*. K. T. Kernan, ed. Los Angeles: University of California.

Brown v. Board of Education. 1954. 347 U.S. 483, 74 S. Ct. 686, 98 L. Ed. 873.

Buck, Pearl S. 1950. *The Child Who Never Grew*. New York: Day.

Cleland, Charles C. and Gary Sluyter. 1973. The heterobedfast ward: a model for translating "normalization" into practice. *Mental Retardation*, 11:44–46.

Cohen, Julius S. and Henry DeYoung. 1973. The role of litigation in the improvement of programming for the handicapped. In Lester Mann and David Sabatino, eds., *The First Review of Special Education*, Vol. 2. Philadelphia: Buttonwood Farms.

Cole, M. and K. Traupmann. 1980. *Comparative Cognitive Research from a Learning Disabled Child*. Minneapolis: University of Minnesota Press.

Commonwealth of Massachusetts. 1847. House of Representatives, No. 152. Report in part to the Legislature of Massachusetts by the Commissioners Appointed to Inquire into the Condition of Idiots within the Commonwealth. Boston: Acts and Resolves of the General Court.

1848. Senate Document 51. Report of Commissioners to Inquire into the Conditions of Idiots of the Commonwealth of Massachusetts. Boston: Acts and Resolves of the General Court.

1850. Senate 38. Report of Dr. S. G. Howe on "Training and Teaching Idiots" under Resolves of April 8, 1848. Boston: Acts and Resolves of the General Court.

1850. Chapter 150. An Act To Incorporate the Massachusetts School for Idiotic and Feebleminded Youth. Boston: Acts and Resolves of the General Court.

1886. Chapter 298. An Act Concerning the Massachusetts School for the Feebleminded. Boston: Acts and Resolves of the General Court.

1972. Chapter 766. An Act Further Regulating Programs for Children Requiring Special Education and Providing Reimbursement Therefor. Boston: Acts and Resolves of the General Court.

Council for Exceptional Children. 1975. What is mainstreaming? *Exceptional Children*, 42:174.

Curtis, W. Scott. 1975a. Adjustment of deaf–blind children. *Education of the Visually Handicapped*, 7:21–26.

1975b. Learning behavior of deaf–blind children. *Education of the Visually Handicapped*, 7:40–48.

Dailey, Wayne F. *et al.* 1974. Attendant behavior and attitudes toward institutionalized retarded children. *American Journal of Mental Deficiency*, 78: 584–591.

Davis, K. V. *et al.* 1969. Stereotyped behavior and activity level in severe retardates: the effects of drugs. *American Journal of Mental Deficiency*, 73:721–727.

Deacon, Joseph J. 1974. *Joey*. New York: Scribner.

De Grandpre, Bernard. 1973. The Culture of a State Ward. Unpublished Ph.D dissertation, Syracuse University.

Dentler, Robert and Bernard Mackler. 1961. The socialization of retarded children in an institution. *Journal of Health and Behavior*, 2:243–252.

Diana v. Board of Education. 1970. Civil Action No. C–70–37 (N.D. Cal).

Diesing, Paul. 1971. *Patterns of Discovery in the Social Sciences*. New York: Aldine.

Doll, E. A. 1916. Anthropometry as an Aid to Mental Diagnosis: A Simple Method for the Examination of Subnormals. Unpublished Master's thesis, New York University. Vineland, New Jersey: Training School.

  1983. Deborah Kallikak: 1889–1978, A Memorial. *Mental Retardation*, 21:30–32.

Dugdale, R. L. 1877. *"The Jukes" A Study in Crime, Pauperism, Disease and Heredity also Further Studies of Criminals*. New York: G. P. Putnam.

Edelsky, Carole and Teresa Rosegrant. 1980. *Interactions with handicapped children: Who's handicapped?* Austin: Southwest Educational Development Laboratory.

Edgerton, Robert B. 1963. A patient elite: ethnography in a hospital for the mentally retarded. *American Journal of Mental Deficiency*, 68:372–85.

  1967. *The Cloak of Competence*. Berkeley: University of California Press.

  1984. The participant observer approach to research in mental retardation. *American Journal of Mental Deficiency*, 88:498–505.

Edgerton, Robert B. and S. M. Bercovici. 1976. The cloak of competence: years later. *American Journal of Mental Deficiency*, 80:485–497.

Edgerton, Robert B., et al. 1984. The cloak of competence: after two decades. *American Journal of Mental Deficiency*, 88:345–351.

Estes, W. K. 1970. *Learning Theory and Mental Development*. New York: Academic.

Featherstone, Helen. 1981. *A Difference in The Family*. New York: Penguin.

Fernald, Walter E. 1896. Some methods employed in the care and the training of feeble-minded children of the lower grades. *Forty-eighth Annual Report of the Trustees of the Massachusetts School for the Feeble-minded at Waltham, Year ending 1895*. Boston: Wright and Potter.

  1917. *Standardized Fields of Inquiry for Clinical Studies of Borderline Defectives*. New York: National Committee for Mental Hygiene.

Fernald, Walter E. et al. 1918. *Waverley Researchers in the Pathology of the Feeble-minded* (Research Series, Cases 1–10). Memoirs of the American Academy of Arts and Sciences.

Firth, Raymond. 1951. *Elements of Social Organization*. Boston: Beacon.

Ford, Gerald. 1976. Nondiscrimination With Respect to the Handicapped In Federally Assisted Programs, April 26, 1976. Executive Order 111914. Federal Register 41:84.

Foucault, Michel. 1975. *The Birth of the Clinic*. New York: Pantheon.

  1976. *Mental Illness and Psychology*. New York: Harper.

Bibliography

Fuller, P. R. 1949. Operant conditioning of a vegetative human organism. *American Journal of Psychology*, 62:587–599.

Glaser, Barney G. and Anselm Strauss. 1967. *The Discovery of Grounded Theory*. Hawthorne, New York: Aldine.

Gleason, John J. 1981. How am I like those whom I observe? The problem of ethnographer as native in his native land. Paper at the Ethnography in Education Research Forum, University of Pennsylvania, Philadelphia, March 20–22.

1982a. Culture: A view from the inside. Working Papers in Anthropology. New York: Wenner-Gren Foundation.

1982b. The skill of observation and competence in context. Paper at the Annual Meetings of the American Academy on Mental Retardation, Boston, May 31.

Goddard, Henry. 1912. *The Kallikak Family*. New York: Macmillan.

Goffman, Erving. 1961. *Asylums*. Garden City, New York: Anchor Books.

1963. *Stigma*. Englewood Cliffs: Prentice-Hall.

1967. The moral career of the mental patient. In J. G. Manis and B. N. Meltzer, eds., *Symbolic Interaction*. Boston: Allyn and Bacon.

Gombrich, E. H. 1972. *Art and Illusion*. Princeton: Princeton University Press.

1979. *The Sense of Order*. Ithaca: Cornell University Press.

Goode, David A. 1974. Some aspects of interaction among congenitally blind deaf and normal persons. Paper, Departments of Sociology and Psychiatry, University of California at Los Angeles.

1975a. Some aspects of embodied activity on a deaf blind, retarded ward in a state hospital. Paper, Departments of Sociology and Psychiatry, University of California at Los Angeles.

1975b. Some procedures for locating competence in the congenitally deaf-blind retarded: towards the grounds for achieving human intersubjectivity. Mental Retardation Research Center: University of California.

1980a. Behavioral sculpting: parent-child interactions in families with retarded children. In J. Jacobs, ed. *Mental Retardation*. Springfield, Illinois: Thomas.

1980b. The world of the congenitally deaf blind: towards the grounds for achieving human understanding. In J. Jacobs, ed., *Mental Retardation*. Springfield, Illinois: Thomas.

Goode, David A. and Michael R. Gaddy. 1976. Ascertaining choice with alingual, deaf-blind and retarded clients. *Mental Retardation*, 14:10–12.

Gorton, Chester and John Hollis. 1965. Redesigning a cottage unit for better programming and research for the severely retarded. *Mental Retardation*, 3:16–21.

Gould, Stephen Jay. 1981. *The Mismeasure of Man*. New York: Norton.

Greenfield, J. 1965. *A Child Called Noah*. New York: Holt, Rinehart and Winston.

1978. *A Place for Noah*. New York: Holt, Rinehart and Winston.

Greenspan, S. 1979. Social intelligence in the retarded. In N. R. Ellis, ed.,

Bibliography

Handbook of Mental Deficiency. Hillsdale, New Jersey: Lawrence Erlbaum.

Grossman, Herbert J. 1983. *Manual on Terminology and Classification in Mental Retardation*. Washington, D.C.: American Association on Mental Deficiency.

Harmatz, Morton G. 1973. Observational study of ward staff behavior. *Exceptional Children*, 39:554–558.

Harris, John M. *et al.* 1974. Aide–resident ratio and ward population density as mediators of social interaction. *American Journal of Mental Deficiency*, 79:320–326.

Haynes, Sondra. 1973. Change in a State School. Unpublished Ph.D. dissertation, Syracuse University.

Heber, Rick. 1961. *A Manual on Terminology and Classification in Mental Retardation*. Monograph Supplement to American Journal of Mental Deficiency. Washington, D.C.: American Association of Mental Deficiency.

Hermanson, Colleen and J. P. Das. 1977. Social interaction between caregivers and profoundly retarded children. *Mental Retardation Bulletin*, 5:101–114.

Higgins, Jean C. 1970. *Lindy*. Valley Forge, Pennsylvania: Judson.

Hirsch, Ernest. 1959. The adaptive significance of commonly described behavior of mentally retarded. *American Journal of Mental Deficiency*, 63:639–646.

Hobson v. Hansen. 1967. 269 F. Supp. 401 (D.D.C. 1967), cert. denied, aff'd sub. nom., 393 U.S. 801, 89 S. Ct. 40, 21 L. Ed. 2d 85.

Hobson v. Hansen–II. 1971. 320 F. Supp. 720 (D.D.C. 1971).

Hollis, John H. 1976. Steady transition states: Effects of alternative activity on body-rocking in retarded children. *Psychological Reports*, 39:91–104.

Howe, Samuel G. 1847. Fieldnotes on and of Observations made [of] Idiotic Persons In the Commonwealth of Massachusetts. Unpublished notebook. Waltham, Massachusetts: Fernald State School for the Mentally Retarded.

———. 1853. Fifth Annual Report of the Massachusetts School for Idiots and Feebleminded Youth, 1852. Cambridge: Metcalf.

———. 1870. Twenty-Second Annual Report of the Trustees of the Massachusetts School for Idiotic and Feebleminded Youth, 1869. Boston: Wright and Potter.

———. 1875. Twenty-Seventh Annual Report of the Trustees of the Massachusetts School for Idiotic and Feebleminded Youth, 1874. Boston: Wright and Potter.

———. 1876. Twenty-Eighth Annual Report of the Trustees of the Massachusetts School for Idiotic and Feebleminded Youth, 1875. Boston: Wright and Potter.

Hrdlicka, Ales. 1898. Report on anthropological work in the State Institution for Feebleminded Children, Syracuse, New York. In *Forty-Eighth Annual Report of the Managers of the Syracuse State Institution for Feebleminded Children, 1898*. New York: Wynkoop Hallenback Crawford.

Hunt, Nigel. 1967. *The World of Nigel Hunt: The Diary of a Mongoloid Youth*. Beaconsfield: Finlayson.

Bibliography

Itard, Jean-Marc-Gaspard. 1962. *The Wild Boy of Aveyron*. New York: Appleton-Century-Crofts.

Izutsu, S. 1971. A motivation and training program for the severely and profoundly mentally retarded. Conference on Occupational Therapy for the Multiply Handicapped Child, 1971. W. L. West, ed. 278–321.

Jacobs, Jerry, ed. 1980. *Mental Retardation*. Springfield, Illinois: Thomas.

Johnstone, E. R. 1923. *Dear Robinson*. Vineland: Smith.

Kaufman, M. E. and H. Levitt. 1965. Some determinants of stereotyped behaviors in the institutionalized mental defectives. *Journal of Mental Deficiency Research*, 9:201–209.

Kaufman, Sandra Z. 1980. *Research in Progress: A retarded daughter educates her mother*. Keith T. Kernan, ed. Los Angeles: University of California.

Kernan, Keith T. and Paul Koegel. 1980. *Employment Experiences of Community Based Mildly Retarded Adults*. L. L. Langness, ed. Los Angeles: University of California.

Kernan, Keith T. and Sharon Sabsay. 1979. *Semantic deficiencies in the narratives of mildly retarded speakers*. L. L. Langness, ed. Los Angeles: University of California.

1982. *Getting there: Directions given by mildly retarded and non retarded adults*. K. T. Kernan, ed. Los Angeles: University of California.

Killian, E. W. 1967. *New approaches to teaching children hitherto crucial crib cases*. Denver: A paper at the American Association of Mental Deficiency.

Koegel, Paul. 1978. *The Creation of Incompetence*. L. L. Langness, ed. Los Angeles: University of California.

Koegel, Paul and Keith Kernan. 1980. *Issues Affecting The Involvement of Mildly Retarded Individuals in Competitive Employment*. Los Angeles: University of California.

Kroeber, A. L. and Clyde Kluckhohn. 1952. Culture. Papers of the Peabody Museum of American Archaeology and Ethnology. Vol. 47. Cambridge, Mass.: Peabody Museum, Harvard University.

Landesman-Dwyer, S. 1974. A description and modification of the behavior of the non-ambulatory, profoundly mentally retarded children. Unpublished Ph.D. dissertation, University of Washington.

Lane, Harlan. 1979. *The Wild Boy of Aveyron*. Cambridge, Mass.: Harvard University Press.

Langness, L. L. 1965. *The Life History in Anthropological Science*. New York: Holt, Rinehart and Winston.

1982. Mental Retardation as an Anthropological Problem. The Wenner-Gren Foundation Working Paper Series on the Anthropology of the Handicapped. New York: Wenner-Gren Foundation.

Langness, L. L. and Gelya Frank. 1981. *Lives*. San Francisco: Chandler and Sharp.

Langness, L. L. and Levine, Harold G., eds. 1986. *Culture and Retardation*. Boston: Reidel.

Lederman, S. J. 1969. Behavioral and heartrate responses to visual stimuli in profoundly retarded children. Unpublished Master's Thesis, University of Wisconsin.

Bibliography

Levine, Harold G. and L. L. Langness. 1983. Context, ability, and performance: comparison of competitive athletics among mildly mentally retarded and non retarded adults. *Journal of Mental Deficiency*, 87:528–538.

Levy, Ellen and William Mcleod. 1977. The effects of environmental design on adolescents in an institution. *Mental Retardation*, 15:28–32.

Lewis, E. O. 1933. Types of mental deficiency and their social significance. *Journal of Mental Science*, 79:298–304.

Longhurst, T. M. 1972. Assessing and increasing descriptive communication skills in retarded children. *Mental Retardation*, 19:42–45.

   1974. Communication in retarded adolescents: sex and intelligence level. *American Journal of Mental Deficiency*, 78:607–618.

MacAndrew, C. and R. B. Edgerton. 1964. The everyday life of institutionalized idiots. *Human Organization*, 23:312–318.

MacMillan, D. 1977. *Mental Retardation in School and Society*. Boston: Little, Brown.

Mann, Lester and David A. Sabatino, eds. 1973. *The First Review of Special Education*. Philadelphia: Buttonwood Farms.

Mercer, Jane R. 1973. *Labeling the Mentally Retarded*. Berkeley: University of California Press.

Meyers, C. Edward. 1978. *Quality of Life in Severely and Profoundly Mentally Retarded People*. Washington: American Association on Mental Deficiency.

Mills v. Board of Education of the District of Columbia. 1971. Civil Action No. 1939–71 (D.D.C. 1971).

Montessori, Maria. 1912. *The Montessori Method*. New York: Pantheon.

   1913. *Pedagogical Anthropology*. New York: Stokes.

Murray, Dorothy. 1967. *This is Stevie's Story*. New York: Abingdon.

National Association of Superintendents of Public Residential Facilities for the Mentally Retarded. 1974. *Residential Programming*. Washington, D.C.: President's Committee on Mental Retardation.

National Institute on Mental Retardation. 1978. *Residential Services*. Canadian Association for the Mentally Retarded.

New York State Association for Retarded Children, Inc. v. Rockefeller. 1972. U.S. District Court, E.D.N.Y.

O'Brien, John and Coonie Poole. n.d. *Planning Spaces*. Atlanta, Georgia: Georgia Association for Retarded Citizens.

O'Donnel, Brigid. 1976. Resident rights interview. *Mental Retardation*, 14:13–17.

Paul, James L. *et al.* 1977. *Deinstitutionalization*. Syracuse: Syracuse University.

Pennsylvania Association for Retarded Children v. Commonwealth of Pennsylvania. 1971. Civil Action No. 71–42 (E.D. Pa. 1971).

Pinel, Philippe. 1962. A treatise on insanity. In *The History of Medicine* Vol. 5. New York: Hafner.

Piper, T. J. and R. C. MacKinnon. 1969. Operant conditioning of a profoundly retarded individual reinforced via a stomach fistula. *American Journal of Mental Deficiency*, 73:627–630.

Bibliography

Price-Williams, Douglass and Sharon Sabsay. 1979. Communicative
competence among severely retarded persons. *Semiotica*, 26:35–63.

Public Law 89–97. 1965. Social Security Amendments. U.S. Statutes-at-Large,
79:286–423.

Public Law 94–142. 1976. Education of the Handicapped Act. Washington:
Government Printing Office.

Rago, William. 1976. Teritoriality. Unpublished Ph.D. dissertation, University
of Texas, Austin.

   1977a. Eye gaze and dominance hierarchy in profoundly mentally retarded
   males. *American Journal of Mental Deficiency*, 82:145–148.

   1977b. Identifying profoundly mentally retarded subtypes as a means of
   institutional grouping. *American Journal of Mental Deficiency*. 8:470–473.

Rehabilitation Act. 1973. Section 504 (29 U.S.C. 794).

Reynolds, Maynard. 1967. Hierarchy of Special Education Services. Council for
Exceptional Children Convention, New York.

Rhodes, William C. and Sabin Head. 1974. *A Study of Child Variance:
Conceptual Project in Emotional Disturbance. Vol. III: Service Delivery
Systems.* Ann Arbor: University of Michigan.

Rhodes, William C. and Michael Tracy. 1975. *A Study of Child Variance:
Conceptual Project in Emotional Disturbance. Vol. I: Conceptual Models.*
Ann Arbor: University of Michigan.

Ricci v. Greenblat. 1972. Civil Action No. 72–496F (E. D. Mass. 1972).

Rice, H. K. 1968. Operant behavior in vegetant patients. *Psychological Record*,
18:297–302.

Rice, H. K. and M. W. McDaniel. 1966. Operant behavior in vegetative
patients. *Psychological Record*, 16:279–281.

Rice, H. K., et al. 1967. Operant behavior in vegetative patients, II.
Psychological Record, 17:449–460.

Roberts, Nancy and Bruce Roberts. 1962. *One of Those Children*. New York:
Taplinger.

Rogers, A. C. and Maud A. Merrill. 1919. *Dwellers in the Vale of Siddem*.
Boston: Badger.

Rogers, Warren and Ann and Donald Baer. 1976. An Analysis of Two
Naturally Covarying Behaviors. Unpublished paper, American
Psychological Association, Washington, D.C.

Rueda, Robert. 1982. *Communicative and Social Competence*. Manuscript
Laboratory of Comparative Human Cognition. Cambridge, Mass.:
Harvard University.

Rueda, Robert and K. Chan. 1980. Referential communication skills of
moderately mentally retarded adolescents. *American Journal of Mental
Deficiency*, 85:45–52.

Ryle, Gilbert. 1971. *Collected Essays, 1919–1968* Vol. 1. London:
Hutchinson.

Sackett, Gene. 1978a. *Data Collection and Analysis Methods*. Vol. 2 of
Observing Behavior. 2 vols. Baltimore: University Park Press.

   1978b. *Theory and Applications in Mental Retardation*, vol. 1 of *Observing
   Behavior*. 2 vols. Baltimore: University Park Press.

Bibliography

Scheerenberger, R. C. 1983. *A History of Mental Retardation*. Baltimore: Brookes.

Scott, Curtis W., *et al.* 1975. Learning behavior of deaf-blind children. *Education of the Visually Handicapped*, 7:40–48.

Séguin, Edouard. 1866. *Idiocy and Its Treatment by the Physiological Method.* New York: Wood.

1870. New facts and remarks concerning idiocy. A Lecture Delivered Before the New York Medical Journal Association, October 15, 1869. New York: Wood.

1880. *Report on Education*. Milwaukee: Doerflinger.

1970. *Idiocy*. New York: Columbia University.

Shelton, J. T. *et al.* 1965. Lack of a patient elite: ethnography in a hospital for the mentally retarded. *American Journal of Mental Deficiency*, 70:389–392.

Simeonson, R. J. 1979. Social competence. In *Mental Retardation and Development Disabilities*. J. Wortis, ed. New York: Brunner Mazel.

Sternberg, Les and Gary L. Adams. 1982. *Educating Severely and Profoundly Handicapped Students*. Rockville: Aspen.

Talbot, Mabel E. 1966. *Edouard Séguin*. New York: Teachers College Press.

Taylor, Steven J. 1973. Attendants Perspectives: A view from the back ward. Unpublished paper, 97th Annual Meeting of the American Association of Mental Deficiency.

Taylor, Steven, *et al.* 1981. *Title XIX and Deinstitutionalization*. Syracuse: Human Policy Press.

Terman, Lewis. 1916. *The Measurement of Intelligence*. Cambridge, Mass.: Riverside.

Thompson, Travis and John Grabowski. 1977. *Behavior Modification of the Mentally Retarded*. New York: Oxford University Press.

Tizard, Jack. 1970. The role of social institutions in the cause, prevention, and alleviation of mental retardation. In H. S. Haywood, ed., *Social-Cultural Aspects of Mental Retardation*. New York: Appleton-Century-Crofts.

Tizard, Jack and Barbara Tizard. 1974. The Institution as an Environment for Development. In *The Integration of a Child Into A Social World*. New York: Cambridge University Press.

Towfighy-Hooshyar, Nahid. 1978. Speech Interactions Between Caretakers and Institutionalized Severely Retarded. Unpublished Ph.D. dissertation, Indiana University.

Turner, Jim L. 1980. "Yes, I Am Human": Autobiography of a retarded career. *Journal of Community Psychology*, 8:3–8.

Vail, D. J. 1967. *Dehumanization and the Institutional Career*. Springfield, Illinois: Thomas.

Wharton, Noel. 1972. A study of the social functioning of institutionalized mentally retarded crib patients. *Sociological Focus*, 5:120–141.

Whittemore, Robert D. *et al.* 1980. *The Life History Approach to Mental Retardation*. L. L. Langness, ed. Los Angeles: University of California.

Wills, Richard H. 1971. The Institutionalized Severely Retarded. Unpublished Ph.D. dissertation, Northwestern University.

Bibliography

1973. *The Institutionalized Severely Mentally Retarded.* Springfield, Illinois: Thomas.

Winship, A. E. 1900. *Jukes-Edwards.* Harrisburg: Meyers.

Wolfensberger, Wolf. 1972. *Normalization.* Toronto: National Institute on Mental Retardation.

1975. *The Origin and Nature of Institutional Models.* Syracuse: Human Policy.

Wyatt v. Stickney. 1971. 325 F. Supp. 781 (M.D. Ala. 1971).

1972a. Interim Emergency Order (March 2, 1972).

1972b. Order and Decree (April 13, 1972).

Zober, Mark A. 1979. Measuring the impact of social physical environmental characteristics within residential settings on selected adaptive and maladaptive behaviors of institutionalized retarded adults. Unpublished Ph.D. dissertation, Florence Heller Graduate School for Advanced Studies in Social Welfare, Brandeis University.

Index

LaVergne, TN USA
04 January 2011
210930LV00005B/19/P